THE DOCTORS' CLINIC-30 PROGRAM

"A HEALTHY AND EXCITING WEIGHT-LOSS PROGRAM THAT ALLOWS YOU TO EAT PLENTY OF NUTRITIOUS FOOD WITHOUT THE FRUSTRATION OF DIETING."

FOURTH EDITION

BY

J.T. Cooper, M.D., M.P.H.

Eddie Fatakhov, M.D., M.B.A.

Sharon M. Cooper, R.N., M.S.N.

JT Cooper, P.C.
1234 Powers Ferry Road, Suite 104
Marietta, GA 30067
Office: 770-952-7681
Fax: 770-952-8688

www.dietdrtom.com
www.drfatakhov.com
facebook.com/fatakhov
twitter.com/eddiefatakhov

Project Credits:
Senior Editor: Olga Izmaylova
Proofreader: Olga Izmaylova
Assistant Editor: Bhavi Patel
Computer Support: Alexander Neverov

Manufactured in the United States of America

Fourth Edition

DEDICATIONS

This book is dedicated to the late Dr. Tom Cooper, who was truly a remarkable man, and a pioneer in the field of bariatric medicine. He was the past president of the American Society of Bariatric Physicians and the first physician to open a bariatric practice in the State of Georgia. Dr. Cooper spent his whole life developing a unique method for approaching weight loss. He used a combination of science, medicine, psychology, and compassion to bring his patients great success in their weight loss goals. Dr. Cooper spoke seven languages and was an author of eleven books on dieting and nutrition, including the prior editions of The Doctors' Clinic-30 Program. Dr. Cooper was also a contributing author for a textbook on the treatment of obesity, published this year. He was a flight surgeon in the Air Force Reserves and retired as a full Colonel. He will be forever remembered by his patients, family, and through the accomplishments he left behind.

- Sharon Cooper

I would like to dedicate this book to my mother. She is the greatest inspiration in my life, and has really provided her support for me every step of the way.

- Eddie Fatakhov, M.D.

CONTENTS

ACKNOWLEDGEMENTS

I would like to thank all the people in my life, who have helped me along the way, to get this book updated. I would like to first thank my co-author Sharon Cooper, who has provided me with great insight and ideas for this book. This project would not have been a reality without you and all of your help. Thank you.
I would also like to thank Olga Izmaylova for her patience and endless nights reading early manuscripts and making helpful suggestions. In addition I would like to thank Bhavi Patel for her great editorial assistance. Lastly, I would like to thank all my patients, throughout the years, for their words of encouragement and their success stories, which have inspired me to strive for excellence in this constantly evolving field of medicine.

         -    Eddie Fatakhov, M.D.

INTRODUCTION

A PERSONAL MESSAGE FROM THE AUTHORS

"No disease that can be treated by diet should be treated with any other means." - Maimonides

My weight loss journey began when my first husband left me. He took most of my personal belongings, including my furniture, my share of our savings account, and even the sheets off our bed; and left me a note stating that "the fire has died."

At that time, I was 5'7" and weighed 210 pounds. You would think a nurse could do something about her weight, but I couldn't. I spent $399.95 on a home gym. I tried acupuncture. I tried hypnotism. I tried sixteen different diets and failed at all of them. Let me tell you something - in my opinion, diets didn't work! Period. I tried almost every popular diet you could think of. The problem wasn't losing the weight; it was keeping it off, once I lost it.

I just couldn't go through life starving myself, taking dangerous pills, or drinking those chalky-tasting "shakes" every day. I became nervous, irritable, and hungry. I was constantly hungry, so any little thing would trigger my anger. I was a bear or another "B". Finally, I would binge. It was always the same. I'd buy a box of chocolate-filled donuts, the really good kind. Then I'd drive around in my car with the donuts next to me on the front seat, eating them and listening to Rocket 105.

It was my mother who finally talked me into getting real help. She made an appointment for me with our family doctor. He took my history, listened to my complaints about diets, and then recommended a program that was completely different from anything I'd ever seen before. This wasn't a "diet." It was totally different. It was The Original Clinic-30 Program.

I started the program on May 17th. Within the first four days, I only lost three pounds. I was disappointed. However, during the three weeks that followed, my weight began to drop regularly. Within the next 196 days, I went from 202 to 129 pounds. This may not seem like a lot, but to me, it was a miracle. This was the first time in my life I was able to lose weight — and keep it off!

It worked for me for one simple reason: I was allowed to eat. I was able to eat three delicious meals plus a snack or two, every day, seven days a week. As a result, I wasn't hungry, irritable, or bingeing on donuts; and I was losing weight!

Throughout the years, this program's results have been published in the International Journal of Obesity and other prominent research publications.

Copies of The Original Clinic-30 Program — developed by Dr. Cooper — were provided to senior medical school students, interns, and physicians to determine its effectiveness; so other doctors have tested this program. Until Dr. Cooper authorized Green Tree Press to publish The Clinic-30 Program in the early 1990s, it was only available to physicians and no one else. Today, with the Internet and E-Books being so popular, it is a lot easier to make this program available to the general public.

With this program, you will be able to enjoy all of your favorite foods, such as meat, chicken, fish, fruits, vegetables, potatoes, pasta, soups, baked goods, sauces, and great-tasting snacks. You'll also enjoy the variety; there are literally hundreds of selections and combinations to choose from. Some are gourmet meals; others are simple soups and sandwiches.

Best of all, the program is easy-to-follow because you don't have to count calories or keep diaries. There are no special foods to buy; everything is available at your local supermarket. There are no pills, powders, artificial foods, drugs, or "strange" foods. Everything is explained on a day-by-day basis.

I wish you the best.

- Sharon Cooper, R.N., M.S.N.

A MESSAGE FROM DR. COOPER

I used to be really heavy. At one point, I actually belonged to "Overeaters Anonymous". I know you are seeking a program that works; a program you can enjoy without feeling deprived.

I'm sure you're wondering, "How can a person eat a lot and still lose weight?" The secret is not in the amount of food you eat; it is in the types of food you eat. The following chapters will detail prescribed combinations of specific foods (such as nutritionally dense special fibers, unrefined carbohydrates, and certain proteins) you should be eating throughout each 24-hour period.

So, how does this program work? In The Doctors' Clinic-30 Program, there are certain foods that will be able to create "the thermic effect". In laymen's terms, it means that specific combinations and selections of food will amplify and extend your metabolism. Therefore, calories are burned more consistently, not just in spurts, like many other diets you may have previously tried.

Everyone is familiar with prescription "diet pills". Well, The Clinic-30 Program actually incorporates many of the same benefits those pills provide, but without the adverse side effects.

My patients, who have tried the program, have more energy, more vitality, and a reduced craving for food. They also enjoy an increase in the serotonin level, which decreases your anxiety, while brightening and uplifting your spirits. Finally, my patients experience a secondary surge in metabolism. That, together with the thermic effect of the foods, allows them to eat more frequently — and still lose weight!

One of my patients was almost arrested because she lost 73 pounds. She was stopped near Sandy Springs, an Atlanta suburb, and was almost taken in to the police station because her driver's license picture didn't look like her any more. Another patient told me how her self-esteem improved after she lost weight and she, now, loves to ambush her husband with hugs and kisses. For some patients, revenge is the motive. One of my patients told me her husband abandoned her and she lost over 60 pounds after their divorce. Now, she teases her ex-husband with her succession of "hunks", whom she parades in front of him and his friends. Revenge is sweet, indeed!

Those success stories, plus the wide variety of letters from people who purchased the program through Green Tree Press, Inc., illustrate its unique effectiveness. The Doctors' Clinic-30 Program can radically change your life. If you follow this program, you can live a healthier, happier life. You will decrease your risk for certain diseases, caused by excess weight, and you will improve your overall quality of life.

That might sound like a big order, but I think you'll agree that excess weight leads to numerous health problems, over time. You want to change that. That's why you're looking at The Doctors' Clinic-30 Program. Good. You're on the right track. You've taken the first step. I won't let you down. I want to help you by sharing the knowledge I've gained over the past 35 years as a medical doctor, specializing in the field of bariatric medicine (the medical management of obesity).

The knowledge contained in this book comes from hundreds of sources in academic and clinical research on obesity, and from my experience in treating thousands of patients with weight problems. I've consulted articles and publications written by top researchers and clinicians in bariatric medicine, in order to provide you the very latest information on how to lose weight, and how to keep it off forever.

Specifically, I would like to thank Dr. Judith Wurtman of Massachusetts Institute of Technology. Dr. Albert Stunkard, Dr. George Bray, Dr. George Blackburn, Dr. Bruce Bistrian, Dr. Bill Asher, Dr. Dal Baker, Dr. Ray Dietz, Dr. Pi-Sunyer, and the late Dr. Peter Lindner.

- J.T. Cooper, M.D.

A MESSAGE FROM DR. FATAKHOV

I am currently a physician at Georgia Regents Medical Center. I have a Bachelor's Degree in Nutrition, with a minor in Sports Wellness. Prior to medical school, I was a personal trainer for six years.

When I was asked to co-author the fourth edition of the Doctors' Clinic-30 Program, I was extremely honored; I gained an opportunity to edit a book written by Dr. Cooper, one of the pioneers in bariatric medicine. This book is not about fad diets or quick weight loss plans. This is a program that provides the tools for a healthy, sustainable weight loss; it is about changing your life-style.

Throughout the years, I trained clients of all ages, weight, and body type. As a nutritionist, I created meal plans for a vast number of people. Now, as a physician, I treat numerous patients, daily. I noticed that a lot of my former clients and patients had a similar problem – obesity. And, as a result of their obesity, they developed diabetes, hypertension, and obstructive sleep apnea. I believe that every single one of those patients would benefit greatly from this program.

Obesity is a real problem and it is not going away anytime soon. The Doctors' Clinic-30 Program is instrumental to battling our nation's obesity problem. Instead of providing another diet plan, this program is based on change and lifestyle modification. After all, a diet is just a temporary measure; people always diet with a specific goal and time limit in mind. For example, a person going to the beach will diet for a few months prior to the trip, but upon return will quit dieting and gain the weight back. This program strives to avoid the constant back-and-forth by providing you with the tools you need to lose weight and keep it off; it focuses on maintaining good nutrition and eating habits over a lifetime.

The Coopers were ahead of their time when they wrote the first edition of this book in the early 1990s; it became quite popular during the Weight Watchers era. This book explains the exchange system (used by Weight Watchers) and describes an easy and healthy way to lose weight, without counting calories, downloading fancy apps, or keeping food journals.

Additionally, this book includes many recipes, which are culturally diverse. As a Russian native, there are many dishes I enjoy and would not want to give up for a diet. Luckily, this book incorporates recipes from all over the world; for example, a recipe for Borscht, a Russian beet-based soup, is included. This program prepares you for a lifetime commitment to healthy eating, and allows you to eat the food you love and lose weight, simultaneously.

Once you are done with this program, I guarantee you will have more energy, feel great, and decrease the physical harms of being overweight. Most importantly, you will lose weight and have all the knowledge and tools to keep it off.

- Eddie Fatakhov, M.D.

PRAISES WITHIN

Here are several comments from people who purchased The Doctors' Clinic-30 Program over the years.

Kitty R. wrote to say she lost 56 pounds:

"The Clinic-30 Program works! I'm an example. What I like best is that I can eat a lot and still lose weight! I recommended it to a couple of friends and they started losing weight, too!"

Anne G., High Point, NC writes:

"I lost 25 lbs. in two months. I talk about it so much that others in my workplace have bought their own programs."

Melissa Daniels wrote:

"I was very successful...I lost over 100pounds."

Beth Shaw told us:

"We followed the program and my husband lost over 100 pounds!"

Steven R. wanted to buy two-dozen copies:

"My weight was 194 lbs., now it is 157 lbs. My wife was 159 lbs., now she weighs 133 lbs. My daughter was 175 lbs., now she weighs 150 lbs....our neighbors all want to know where to get the program...is it possible to send me two dozen?"

Samantha E., Lake Leure, NC:

"This is the best plan I have ever tried. It works! I lost 10 lbs. in a month and I was always eating. I am excited and feel so good! I am ordering these for my mother, daughter, and sister—please send them as soon as

possible. Thank you, thank you."

Frances M., Memphis, TN:

"I did not believe it...but it works. Every diet I've ever tried, every diet pill, liquid, or fad did not work. But with The Clinic-30, I lost 28 lbs. in about 2 months. It's great to be able to keep it off. I've loaned it to several people — but have a hard time getting it back."

Kathleen H., Huntington Station, NY:

"I've been on The Doctors' Clinic-30 for about 6 weeks. I have lost 20 pounds and 4.5 inches from my waistline. This may not seem world-shaking to some people, but this is from someone who gained weight on every other program I tried. I have never been hungry...there is so much variety. I have three friends on your program now."

Heidi E., Zephyrhills, FL:

"I started my husband on the program March 24th and, to date, he has lost twelve pounds. He is having knee surgery on June 5th, so it was essential he lost weight. All of our other diets failed, but this one is working. Funny thing, I found out I lost five pounds also!"

Gilman D., Sturgeon Falls, Ontario:

"This program has really worked for my wife and I. Between the two of us we lost a total of 150 pounds! Thank you for making such a wonderful program accessible to the public."

Singe M., San Francisco, CA:

"I am 69 years young, and the weight does not come off easily at this age. BUT I AM THRILLED AT THE RESULTS I HAVE RECEIVED. I am NEVER hungry. I seem to have more food to eat than when I was trying to be careful."

Randi T., Brownville, ME:

"I think your program is wonderful. I went to the doctor to get a checkup. He gave me the okay to begin The Clinic-30 Program. Now my

cholesterol and blood pressure are very good. I'm down to 111 lbs. and feeling great!"

Anne G., High Point, NC:

"I lost 25 lbs. in two months. I talked about it so much in my workplace that others bought their own copies of The Clinic-30 Program. It's like my second Bible. I was even able to keep it off during the holidays. I am so proud of myself and I think I look great in a size 12. Even some size 10's."

Gretchen G., Honolulu, HI:

"I love this program. I'm purchasing another copy for my best friend. As the manager of a recreation center, I put one recipe per week on the fitness room mirror and the responses have been great."

Lonnie T., Voorheesville, NY:

"I have lost 53 lbs. and feel great. Send me 2 more copies of your Clinic-30 Program. I think the program is wonderful!"

Pamela R., Laramie, WY:

"I am so happy that my son has followed The Doctors' Clinic-30 Program and his doctor was so happy with him. He showed the doctor The Clinic-30 Program and the doctor is ordering it. Several of his nurses are going to order the program also. It's simply great!!!! As of this date, Robert lost 50 lbs."

Caroline T., Columbus, GA:

"It's very easy to follow and I eat what I want...nothing frozen...nothing tastes like cardboard. It is absolutely wonderful. Here I am eating all of this food and losing weight. The greatest gift my mother has ever given me is your program. The greatest gift I gave myself was the day I traded my size 18 blue jeans in for a size 14."

CHAPTER ONE

GETTING STARTED ON THE RIGHT FOOT

"Success is what you want, happiness is wanting what you get." - W.P Kinsella

WHY THIS PROGRAM IS DIFFERENT

Diets don't work and they can't work - ever! What does work is an eating program that is sensible, safe, affordable, and easy to follow. The Doctors' Clinic-30 Program is based on sound principles, research, and testimonials from previous patients.

The critical difference in The Doctors' Clinic-30 Program is that it takes into account the fact that we live in a very fast-paced society: Who has a soccer game? Who's in music class? Who's going out for a meeting? Trying to cook and keep track of everybody in the house is a major undertaking. You certainly don't need to spend an additional half-hour or more in the kitchen whipping up special diet foods.

When reading this book, please start at the beginning and read each chapter carefully. Don't jump ahead; there's a chronological order here that's vital to your success. This is a very simple and easy-to-understand program.

This program will show you why most people become overweight and how continuing to stay this way can shorten lives and cause a number of serious health problems. That information is not intended to frighten you. You need to be aware of all the facts and dangers of obesity, so you can make an informed decision on whether starting this program is the right choice for you.

Our inner feelings are important for controlling problem eating. Our past experiences also affect how well we do on a weight control program.

Attitudes of others toward an obese person are often quite interesting and important to know about. These forms of overt and covert sabotage can be devastating to a slimming program, unless the person with the problem can deal with such damaging influences.

You will learn how to deal with saboteurs and how to overcome situations that lead to overeating. This program will teach you how to have positive interactions with your family, friends, co-workers, and significant others. Some of those people, either knowingly or not, can hamper your efforts in losing weight.

Failures in any program can come from overly intricate instructions. The "exchange" plan makes following the important slimming part of this program very simple. It will be explained in more detail in chapter five, but the plan consists of lists of allowable foods from seven food groups, and the amounts you're allowed to eat. The basic food groups will be covered, using a simplified way to keep track of what you eat and what foods are left in the daily allotment in each of the seven food groups. You exchange what you want to eat from each group, knowing how many portions (or "exchanges") you're allowed each day from that group. Below is a checklist of daily portions you will consume from each food group.

DAILY PORTIONS

- Three portions from the bread-starch group
- Three to four portions from the fruit group
- Five portions from the meat and meat-like group
  - Women over 5'10" and all men should consume seven portions
- Four portions from the low-fat or no-fat milk group
  - Includes some soy products for vegetarians
- Two to three portions from the fully cooked vegetable group
- Unlimited raw vegetables from the free vegetable group
- Unlimited salad materials and Super Soup
  - Refer to Chapter 12 for Super Soup Recipe
- Salad dressings and dips – Total of 100 Calories
- Additional free foods

There won't be any calorie counting. You can create your own menu; and, as you can see from the list above, you're allowed ample fruits, vegetables, starches, bread, milk products, salads, and lean protein products. Also, once you reach the maintenance part of the program, you will be provided a list — by brand name — of soups, frozen entrees, and other foods that you can still eat and figure into your exchanges.

This program follows the new guidelines outlined in the 2010 report of the Surgeon General. The program is low in fat and high in natural fiber, fresh fruits and vegetables. Legumes (beans and peas) and the right kinds of bread are also a part of the diet, along with delicious salads that are complemented by low-fat dressings and dips. The content of sugar, saturated fats, cholesterol, and sodium is low enough to meet even the most rigid dietetic standards. There is rarely any true hunger; being on this program is as close to a non-diet as you can get and still be effective.

You must keep an open mind and work hard to change the behavior and bad habits that led to your weight problem. We'll spend considerable time on this in the chapters ahead analyzing obesity, looking at factors that cause it, and ways to overcome those factors. We will also talk about exercises, such as walking, that will help you maintain your weight loss, tone your muscles, and build cardiovascular strength.

I hope you take advantage of this program, attain your goal weight, and maintain it for the rest of your life!

IS THIS PROGRAM RIGHT FOR YOU: A NOTE OF CAUTION

Unfortunately, The Doctors' Clinic-30 Program is not for everyone. If you fall into any of the below-listed categories, please consult your physician prior to beginning this program.

1. People Seeking Quick Weight Loss. Losing a lot of weight in a short amount of time is never healthy. With The Doctors' Clinic-30 Program, the average weight loss, in one month, is somewhere between eight and ten pounds. Please be aware that losing more than ten pounds in one month is not a healthy rate of weight loss. Any program that promises such extreme weight loss is likely detrimental to your health. Prior to starting any weight loss program, always remember to discuss it with your physician.
2. Pregnant or Lactating Women. Prior to beginning this program, make sure you are not pregnant; a good rule of thumb is to wait until the first day of your menstrual flow. Reducing the protein and/or caloric contents of your daily diet below a certain level could result in injury to the fetus. If you become pregnant, after starting the program, please consult with your physician regarding an appropriate diet during your pregnancy.
3. Those Taking Lithium for Control of Certain Psychiatric Illnesses. Chemically, lithium is a first cousin to sodium (salt). This program is designed to help one excrete a lot of salt and water. Controlling lithium levels in the body becomes extremely difficult because lithium is excreted from the body more rapidly during this program.

4.   Those Diagnosed With Diabetes. Diabetics usually have special dietary needs and restrictions. There are several weight loss programs, designed specifically for diabetics. Please consult your physician regarding your weight loss goals and appropriate weight loss programs for you.

5.   Those With Liver or Kidney Problems. People suffering with liver or kidney problems have special dietary needs and restrictions. This program does not account for those specific needs and restrictions. Please consult your physician regarding your dietary needs and restrictions.

6.   Those Taking Coumadin (Warfarin) for Atrial Fibrillation, Clots (DVT/PE), or Those With Genetic Deficiency That Predisposes Them to Develop Clots. This program integrates a lot of green vegetables into the daily meals and recipes. Green vegetables contain Vitamin K, which will make Coumadin (Warfarin) less effective, and could be detrimental to your health. Please consult your physician regarding a weight loss program that is appropriate for you.

CHAPTER TWO

FAT... HOW YOU GOT IT AND WHY IT WON'T GO AWAY

"A healthy outside starts from the inside." –
Robert Urich

Throughout Dr. Cooper's 45 years of experience in the field of bariatric medicine, he discovered that in almost all cases, the onset of obesity followed one or more stressful situations in a person's life. Some of those stressors were surgery, childbirth, marriage, divorce, a new job, emotional trauma, the death of a loved one, or illness. No matter the situation, it was followed by a relentless and constant battle against fat.

Once people put on extra weight, they usually go through a series of diets, weight loss routines, attempts at exercise, and sometimes surgery to "cure" the obesity. The story is usually the same in every case - a temporary weight loss is followed by an eventual regaining of the weight, often more weight than before the diet.

This should tell you something: to control your weight, you're going to have to control your life, your emotions, and your response to stress. Don't blame your weight gain on food. Blame it on yourself.

A few years ago, it was popular to blame weight gain on some physical problem, such as the thyroid gland. The truth is, only a small number of people have a physical reason for obesity.

At one time, giving thyroid medication for obesity seemed logical, but this was when testing procedures were primitive and inaccurate. Now, studies have shown that the excess weight lost while on thyroid medication is usually and primarily lean body tissue (especially protein) and not very much fat. In reality, the glands are rarely the cause of weight problems. A simple blood test can rule hypothyroidism out. Giving thyroid medication without a proper test for the presence of thyroid underactivity is not considered good medicine these days. In some cases, taking thyroid medication can be dangerous.

If glands are not the problem, then overweight people must be gluttons, right? Not at all. Most people with a weight problem eat less, at times, than their thin friends. The problem is, they tend to eat more of certain types of foods, and their sense of being hungry is impaired.

One of my patients complained that life was unfair because she had a weight problem while her thin friends did not. I remarked to her that life isn't always fair and probably never would be. I told her that I had to wear glasses in order to see more than 10 feet in front of me, while my sister has perfect vision. I explained that we have to play the hand we are dealt and make the best of what we have. At least we are alive, although forced to diet. That patient was very upset because I explained this basic law of nature and physiology. The truth sometimes hurts, but it's the truth.

If the energy you eat (calories) equals the energy you expend each day (calories burned), the stored body fat will usually stay the same. Whenever energy output (calories burned) increases over intake (calories consumed), our bodies make up the deficit by tapping the energy in our fat stores, producing weight loss. The opposite occurs when energy intake exceeds output; we deposit a daily amount of extra energy in our fat banks, causing our fat stores to increase.

I told my patient that the secret of all those thin people, who seem to stay the same with ease, is in their activity patterns and the habits they've adopted of only eating when hungry.

That is why your thin friends stay thin.

Thin habit patterns include moving around a lot more than an overweight person does. A thin eating pattern is based mostly on internal signals. Hunger produces an episode of eating to satisfy the needs of the body. "Fullness" stops the eating, even if there's something still left on the plate.

Overweight people are slaves to the external world when it comes to eating. You might eat until the plate or bowl is empty. You might also eat in response to external cues and influences. Emotions cause you to eat as well. It's no accident the so-called "hunger center" in the hypothalamus (a part of the brain) is located quite close to the areas that seem to be the source of strong emotions and feelings.

Well, if hunger is the problem, then won't drugs to reduce the urge to eat solve the problem? No, because true hunger is extremely uncommon in the chronically obese, and the use of a hunger stopper is relatively ineffective in attacking impulse eating. Research has shown that certain medications do exert a positive and beneficial effect on certain cases of obesity, but their indiscriminate use, without a physician's care, should be condemned.

This program teaches you how to lose weight without involving pills.

HOW OBESITY CAN HURT YOU

Being overweight carries significant health risks. In addition to the decreased quality of life, studies show there are increased risks for such diverse problems as coronary artery disease, hypertension and hypertensive heart disease, gallbladder disease, certain types of cancer, arthritis, respiratory diseases, and strokes, just to name a few.

Some risks, such as coronary artery disease, are secondary. In that condition, the elevated blood pressures, increased levels of blood fats, and problems with diminished sugar tolerance increase the risks for heart attack and for death.

According to the Centers for Disease Control and Prevention (CDC), more than one-third of U.S. adults and nearly 17% of children are obese. Obesity has surpassed tobacco as the number one cause of preventable death in the United States. According to the CDC, the annual medical costs for the treatment of obesity in the United States were $200 billion dollars in 2010. Those costs increase every year.

I don't mean to scare you. There's a positive side to all this. The good news is that even modest degrees of weight loss produce marked drops in formerly elevated blood pressures. Part of that may result from eating less salt, but a good part of it has to do with the drop in the fat mass of the body.

Insurance actuaries have shown that a drop in body weight produces a better life expectancy for the obese, as compared to someone who remains fat and does nothing about it.

There's apparently some connection between how the fat is arranged on the body and the incidence of these deadly diseases, particularly heart disease. Those with a so-called "pear shape" obesity have a lot of the fat on the thighs, buttocks, and hips. They often do resemble pears in the initial body contours before losing weight. The "pear shape" obesity is less deadly than the more dangerous "apple shape."

The "apple shape" obesity strikes mostly men, and most of the excess weight is concentrated on the abdomen. (Thus, the person resembles an apple.)

Preliminary studies indicate that men who are overweight have higher risks of developing certain cancers, including cancer of the colon, rectum, and prostate.

Women who are overweight, particularly in certain age groups, are more prone to cancer of the uterus (both the cervix and the uterine lining), as well as of the ovaries.

Those risks make starting a weight loss program even more imperative. Additionally, proper screening for cancer, blood vessel disease, and other preventable and treatable health problems is important for both sexes.

We can reduce the severity and frequency of those killer diseases by doing a few things a little better than we do now. Our own mental attitudes can wreck our self-improvement efforts. We need to get motivated to do helpful things for ourselves.

I'VE DIETED, BUT DIDN'T LOSE ANY WEIGHT

I've heard this comment many, many times in my practice.

The most common cause of discouragement in any weight loss program is lack of weight loss on the scales. I've had women lose two dress sizes in a month, but because they failed to lose weight on the scales, they quit the program.

That doesn't make sense to me, but it happens.

A person who is successfully losing fat every day will begin to shrink in size. As fat is burned, the body must get rid of the waste products (mostly water) through the kidneys. Sometimes, that waste-water is retained for a little while, artificially raising the weight of the person on the scale. Unless you're aware of what is happening, you can lose your motivation and quit the program.

Think of your body as a living "warehouse," one we can weigh on the scales every day. Inside the "warehouse," you've stored fat, protein, water, salt, bone, tissue, and waste products.

Every day of your life, you put in a certain amount of water and get rid of a certain amount. When you burn fat, this fat is changed to water and waste products, and your body, then, excretes these by-products. If you exercise, healthy muscle tissue is built up into what I call "good weight."

All of these items in your "warehouse" affect what you weigh, depending on how much of each is present the very moment you step on a scale. Water retention caused by medications, excess salt intake, hormones, or the menstrual cycle can force the net weight upward - EVEN THOUGH YOU ARE LOSING FAT DURING THIS TIME.

Irregularity can produce a temporary increase in net weight of as much as two to three pounds. A full bladder can also add an extra pound or so. The good weight from muscle tissue growth can add pounds, too.

What does this mean to you when you step on the scale?

You basically have a number given to you by a hunk of metal. (And many times, a home-scale is inaccurate!) If the number is less than before, you have lost "weight" on the scale.

You can usually believe this indicator of progress, but you CANNOT believe it when you have been good and the scale doesn't show it.

Please don't fall into the scale-watcher trap. If you only look at the weight on the scale, you are doomed to fail. Think more about body composition changes than about scale weight.

I addressed this subject before the actual slimming phase of the Doctors' Clinic-30 Program because it is important you don't torpedo your success before you start. Looking at the scale every day has put an end to many diets.

Don't look at the scale right away. (You will later in the program.) Instead, look at the way your clothes fit. Are they looser on you than they were? Are you able to get into things that had become too small for you before you started your fat loss program?

If so, you have lost FAT, and this is the name of the game — fat loss instead of weight loss!

The scales typically lag one to two weeks behind changes in clothing size, so don't give up and stop your diet for the wrong reasons.

Don't be a slave to the scales. On this program, take the time to really observe what is going on in your body. As the fat is burned off, your healthy protein stores are increased, your size shrinks, and you get slimmer and slimmer. Let your clothes be your guide to your fat loss, not the scale.

TESTIMONIAL

Unless you've been to a particular country or experienced a place so completely "foreign" to you, it's impossible to imagine it, to feel it, no matter how well someone describes it to you. That is what it's like to be seriously obese. The millions who don't have a weight issue, and never will, cannot possibly imagine it; no matter how many times they've watched "The Biggest Loser" or read a heartbreaking, humiliating experience about someone suffering from this disease. They seriously will never know.

I could tell I was dangerously heavy again, without ever getting on the scale. The decorative items on top of my dresser upstairs would vibrate and move as I walked across the floor. Going down the steps required holding carefully onto the banister and moving as slow as if I were 40 years older. I was struggling to catch my breath after walking up a standard set of stairs; buying the very limited and usually hideous clothes in the various big and tall stores; catching random strangers staring at me, whispering to someone about me; feeling like a freak, a second rate citizen. I still remember the feeling when my size 54 shorts were very tight.

I hit rock bottom when I weighed 400 pounds. I was wearing 5X shirts and had a 56-inch waist; I was beyond miserable, words cannot even describe. I would walk up stairs like I was 90 years old, holding the banister and getting winded almost immediately. Running anywhere for any length of time was out of the question. Being stared at ALL THE TIME, EVERYWHERE I WENT was just expected. It wasn't "paranoia," I was a spectacle, an embarrassing one. Sleeping through the night was impossible. Trying to fit into one seat on the plane was humiliating. Going anywhere where others were shirtless was unthinkable. When you are seriously obese, you suffer in all aspects of your life: professionally, socially, physically, mentally, and emotionally. Unless you have been there, you just cannot imagine what it feels like. You can watch the popular TV shows, like "Biggest Loser" or "Extreme Weight Loss," and sympathize with the men and women who are struggling, but until you've been there yourself, it's just impossible to describe or understand.

Over the decades, I learned that for so many people food is as much of an addiction as drugs or alcohol; and it is really hard to break free from it. The consequences of food addiction are often as deadly; they just take a little longer to manifest. I learned that the "hot meals" I grew up with in the 60's and 70's and what we THOUGHT we knew about nutrition was all very wrong. I had no idea that I was relying on food to make me feel good when I was sad, lonely, or bored.

I went to a physician, who prescribed me Adipex. Adipex greatly increased my metabolism. The drug helped me lose my first 40 or so pounds in record time. Then, I hit a plateau, a major one. I learned over time that there is no "magic pill," and believe me, there isn't. There are temporary "helpers," but they never last for long. I finally hit that point where I knew I had to do more; a lot more. I started eating cleaner, not *clean, but cleaner. I cut out fast foods, fried foods, and excessive sweets. I still knew very little about proper nutrition and what you have to do, in addition to proper nutrition, to lose all the weight, keep it off, and stay healthy. I started doing cardio, not weights, just low-impact cardio. Over the next year, I lost about 70 to 75 pounds. Then again, I hit another major plateau. The weight just would not drop.*

I decided to hire a personal trainer. I spoke with numerous ones because there are as many personal trainers as there are stars in the sky. Believe me, I was lucky to find one that had real passion, real commitment to helping me. During my search, I learned that you must seek out professionals that have a real passion, a true interest in guiding you. It is critical to find a professional, who knows their business and knows how the human body works; who will help you reach your goals. In my case, this very knowledgeable, focused trainer worked with me for over 14 months. I had been so miserable for so long that I was finally at that place where I could say I was ALL IN. I surrendered to what I knew would be hard, but I had trust in my trainer. I made the conscious decision to do EXACTLY what he said and give my weight loss a fair chance. I decided to stop the excuses and the procrastination, and just try to see if doing this would get me to a HEALTHY weight and positive self-image, both of which I deserved to have. I wanted to be healthy and able to maintain a normal weight, but I knew I had to EARN IT. I simply had to.

The training took 14 months. I had to follow a very simple eating plan; there were no points to count and no binging on "cheat" meals. First, I had to learn to be consistent with my eating; that was the hardest part. Once I mastered eating consistently for a couple of months, it became so easy and routine; it became the "norm." I was eating several meals a day, so I was never hungry. Although the portions were smaller than the "all you can eat" portions I was used to, it was still a lot of food. I ate every 3 hours and drank nothing but water. Because I was ADDICTED to diet sodas and sweet drinks, I thought I would die without them, but once I began drinking only water, it was all I craved. Not to mention, it made me feel incredible. In addition to the clean and consistent eating, I had to do 20 to 40 minutes of cardio after each training session. So four times a week, I would train with free weights and then do my cardio. My trainer mixed up my routines, so they were interesting and new, and my body would not get used to doing the same exercises over and over again. The meal plans would also change, but there was always a mixture of complex carbohydrates and protein, with lots of green vegetables and fruits. I was never hungry. After 14 months of this regimen, I went from 335 pounds and 44% body fat to 220 pounds and 12% body fat. I went from 3XL shirts and 48-inch waist to XL shirts (I am 6'3") and a 34-inch waist.

After being on a consistent eating plan and exercise regimen, it's become the norm. I no longer have to hold on to the banister when I go up the stairs. I'm not winded doing the simplest tasks; I have energy. I can run again. I feel alive and would not trade that feeling for anything, especially not for eating "garbage food that tastes good". I've already lost enough years of my life to refined sugars and unhealthy carbs; they do not control me anymore. I highly recommend The Doctors' Clinic-30 Program to anyone, who is ready to make a change in their eating habits. I am living proof that working hard and eating correctly will bring you the results you desired. The pictures below capture my weight loss progression, as I followed The Doctors' Clinic-30 Program, exercised and received support from my friends and family.

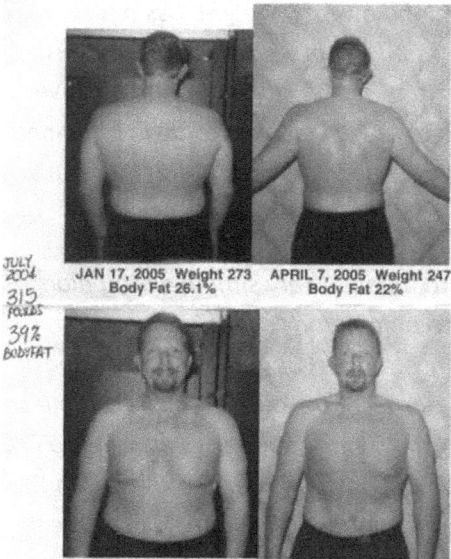

JULY 2004
315 POUNDS
39% BODYFAT

JAN 17, 2005 Weight 273 Body Fat 26.1%   APRIL 7, 2005 Weight 247 Body Fat 22%

CHAPTER THREE

GETTING IN TOUCH WITH YOUR BODY SIGNALS

"With self-discipline, most anything is possible" –
Theodore Roosevelt

Are you hungry right now, as you're reading this?

Do you know what true hunger is, as opposed to false hunger signals?

You might think you know what hunger is, but you don't. The misinterpretation of hunger (or false hunger) is what contributes to present weight problem.

You're reading this now because you have a problem with your weight and eating. For many of you, the thought of being hungry for even a short period of time is frightening.

Let's start with a simple statement that you may dispute, but it has been proven true by some of the best medical and psychological researchers in the world.

MOST PEOPLE WITH A WEIGHT PROBLEM NEVER REALLY FEEL TRUE HUNGER, OR EVEN LACK OF HUNGER.

I'll try to explain that rather surprising statement.

Several well-controlled studies have shown that thin people seem to eat only when hungry. In the study, these slimmer people ate when they were hungry, and refused to eat when hunger was not present. Their internal controls seemed to rule them, as opposed to external cues and influences. You can probably bear this out from your own observations of your thinner friends and acquaintances.

You've observed your thin friends eating much more food than you, including a lot of foods you would not dare eat when trying to lose fat. They do all these seemingly fattening acts, but stay thin.

A thin man or woman may choose to eat chocolate ice cream for lunch and nothing else. He or she may order the most fattening thing on the menu while you eat lettuce and cottage cheese.

These fortunate people are governed by an internal control system that lets them eat what they want, when they want it, and as much as they want. The difference between them and you is that they may eat only two or three bites of ice cream or pastry, and then push the rest away.

You most likely have trouble doing that. I make that assumption because almost all people who are overweight decide when to eat food based on external cues (stress, nervousness, anxiety, etc.) or false internal cues (false hunger pangs).

Just knowing and understanding this goes a long way to helping you understand your own body and its food needs. With this knowledge, you can control when you eat by knowing why you eat.

You might ask, if hunger is the main problem, why not use appetite suppressants to curb hunger pangs?

Like most physicians in private practice, my patients bombard me with requests for "something to kill the appetite."

An appetite suppressant may or may not produce sustained weight and fat loss. It usually doesn't work over a period of time. The weight returns and the patient asks for "something stronger" to help deal with the demands of a weight loss program.

The truth is that "diet pills" can partially control true hunger. The problem is that a person with a weight problem is driven to eat by cues that have nothing to do with true hunger. Diet pills attack the problem from the wrong direction. They should only be taken under a physician's direction, if at all.

Let's look at some of the "hungers" that often plague a patient and ruin a diet program.

When patients come to me with complaints of constant hunger, I ask them to go through certain questions and look internally while doing so.

Ask yourself these same questions:

Are you really hungry? How do you know you feel hunger? Where do you feel the hunger? How long between the times you finished a meal and when you felt hungry? Was the time less than two hours? (If so, the food is still in the process of digesting and is being absorbed into the blood stream even as the "hunger" is being felt). Do you feel any burning, emptiness, growling, spasm, or other uncomfortable feeling in the stomach area? What makes you think the sensations are hunger, instead of the normal contractions of the stomach that follow a few hours after a meal?

Most patients with these hunger pangs find that a dose of antacid or a non-caloric liquid, like water or herbal tea, will usually quiet things down. Instead of a snack that could contain 300-plus calories, the antacid will often stop the discomfort without the penalties of unwanted and unneeded food calories.

If you immediately put food into your stomach whenever it rumbles or burns, then the entire slimming process will be compromised. Remember, hunger suppressants aren't the answer, either. Only with education can a patient be convinced to take antacids or low-calorie soups to ease the discomfort of stress-produced excess acidity and stomach spasms.

Many overweight people have what are called hiatal hernias or weaknesses in the area of the diaphragm where the esophagus passes through on the way to the upper stomach. Back surges of stomach acid can cause distress and a tendency to eat to relieve the pain. Fortunately, the prime treatment for this type of hernia is weight loss, combined with medications to control acid production or neutralize excess acid. If weight is lost, the symptoms get better.

The problem lies in the unknowing patient who treats his or her problem with the very thing that will make it worse — fat-producing excess calories. To avoid the wrong response to what your stomach is "telling" you, the key is to educate yourself.

Whether you call this drive appetite or hunger doesn't matter for now. What is important is to get in touch with your body and mind, and ask both of them some questions every time you feel hunger: Is the food really needed to fuel your body, or are you eating for other reasons?

If you feel hungry during your normal mealtime, then you know that you need to fuel your body. If you feel hungry late at night, an hour after you've eaten or after you had an argument with your spouse, then you probably want to eat for reasons other than hunger.

Emotions and feelings will trigger inappropriate eating, even when a meal has just been eaten and there's no valid reason to eat. We often bury anger, sadness, depression, boredom, frustration, and other strong feelings under a mountain of food. We return almost to infancy, to the thumb in the mouth, the full stomach (along with real or symbolic burping afterwards), the warm and comfortable feeling of oblivion, and the feeling of being loved that comes with being "full" again.

The empty feeling that a lot of problem eaters have may come from excess acid, or it may be a psychological emptiness rather than a real one. I usually remind my patients that the stomach is supposed to be empty most of the time. It's a receptacle and mixing station for foods, not the center of the universe.

I have my patients go through a drill that initially frightens them, but later will give them a certain degree of confidence. I want you to try the same drill.

Eat a good lunch, but don't eat an evening meal or any snacks after noon. You'll not eat again until breakfast the next morning.

You may have all the water and non-caloric beverages that you want, but absolutely no food (not even lettuce).

Have some antacids ready if your stomach starts to rumble or you get "acidy".

During this fast, ask yourself the same questions you asked yourself earlier in this chapter: Are you really hungry? Where do you feel the hunger? Are you sure it's not just acid in your stomach?

When I do this fasting drill in my practice, some people absolutely refuse to go without eating for even that short a time. They are so terrified of doing without food for 18 hours that some have refused, or even quit my program instead of completing the task. For those who complete the semi-fast overnight, there's no question as to the benefit.

I can see a new confidence build in their minds. They find that delaying or skipping a meal or snack is not the ultimate disaster. They don't die and they suffer no ill effects.

This exercise will prepare you for any situation in which you're unable to eat properly — times when you have to delay getting the correct foods; times when you must choose between eating problem or junk foods, or waiting a short time to eat your proper meal. This short exercise is one of the most potent builders of strength in dieting.

Remember, I want you to try it, too.

Another good way to build proficiency and confidence is to write down the favorite food or treat that causes you the most problems. It should be something almost irresistible to you. List the second and third most irresistible items as well.

Now, go buy each item and place a triple portion of each on a plate, in a glass, or in a bowl. The next step is to sit down in front of one or more of these at a time, pick up a spoon or fork, and place one tiny sample into your mouth.

Don't swallow! Hold the sample in the mouth for a full minute by carefully looking at a watch and measuring the time.

Minute up? Good. Now, feel the texture of the food. Let your tongue taste all of the different flavors present. See if you can separate these flavors. After a minute, swallow the portion you placed in your mouth.

Put your fork or spoon down and get up from the table. Let the food sit there for three hours and then place it in the garbage or disposal. Write down your feelings about what you have done with these three favorite foods and answer these questions:

What is it about the food that attracts you so much? Is it your past experiences with the food? Its taste? The full feeling it gives you? The warmth you get from it? Why would you get up at 2 a.m., bundle up, and drive to the convenience store to buy this food?

Now that you understand your craving for this food, ask yourself if there is something else you can substitute for it. If you want something salty and crunchy (like peanuts, potato chips, or popcorn), can you substitute something else, such as celery sticks (which are salty and crunchy)?

How about substituting frozen popsicles made with sugar-free drinks for ice cream? Or using a very thin layer of low-calorie mayonnaise instead of a thick, thick spread of regular mayonnaise?

Make your own substitutions, based on the new knowledge you've gained about your two or three problem foods, the ones that can kill your diet.

Learn to widen the range of foods you eat. Vegetables, salads, soups, and most fruits are almost foreign substances to many problem eaters.

I usually suggest one new food every third day. Eat a new vegetable or fruit over that time. Place the food in your mouth, chew slowly, and savor and analyze the flavors.

If you do this, you will start enjoying foods such as peaches, broccoli, pears, and asparagus.

Trying new foods can relieve boredom, so keep an open mind. Remember, you want to lose weight, and this is one of the steps you must take to reach that goal.

In summary, true hunger is rare. Your body is a storehouse of thousands and thousands of calories of usable energy. The real discomfort we feel when we try to lose weight is in our minds. Getting in touch with your true feelings and learning what the body, mind, and spirit are really saying is the initial goal for all those who want a healthy and slim body.

The keys to permanent weight loss and health are self-knowledge, self-love, self-forgiveness, and self-respect. Attain these and the slim body follows as a natural and comfortably attained result.

CHAPTER FOUR

SHOPPING AND COOKING

"The food you eat can either be the safest and most powerful medicine or the slowest form of poison"-
Ann Wigmore

Before you start the slimming phase of the Doctors' Clinic-30 Program, and before I explain the food charts and exchange system, I want to discuss some important subjects: shopping and cooking.

These are important elements of your weight loss program. Weight loss efforts often fail because people don't shop correctly or don't cook food the right way when they get home.

I promised you wouldn't have to do special cooking, but don't think you're going to be able to deep-fat-fry foods, because you cannot. You have to cut down on fried foods now and for the rest of your life, not only for your weight loss, but also for your health.

That doesn't mean you'll never be able to eat fried foods again. Once you attain your goal weight and go on maintenance, you can eat almost anything (occasionally and in moderate amounts).

HOW TO SURVIVE AT THE GROCERY STORE

The average shopper enters a food store unaware of the multiple influences that shape their buying patterns. The multi-billion-dollar food industry is devoted to making sure you buy certain products, whether you want to or not!

That isn't sinister. The food industry is simply trying to make a profit by selling as much of its products as possible. However, you must learn to sort through the marketing hype and buy only the proper items for your slimming phase, your maintenance program, and the rest of your life. You must also learn to resist impulse buying, which can lead to overeating.

Impulse buying is hard to resist; food companies do everything they can to make you buy their products. Often, supermarkets will saturate the air inside with the odors of food.

One of my earlier experiences as a grocery sack boy, in high school, involved peppermint candy. A candy company brought in massive amounts of peppermint candy puffballs, wrapped in cellophane. There was no odor from the puffballs because they were wrapped; however, the company placed an electric device inside the store that released the odor of peppermint candy.

For the next two weeks, we had record sales of peppermint candy.

Another great example is the mall cookie store or pretzel stand, which can be found at many suburban shopping malls. The odors of freshly baked cookies or pretzels are forced into the mall corridor by a fan, resulting in lots of impulsive cookie and pretzel buying. The odor may either be real or artificially generated, but the results are the same.

See what you're up against?

But do not worry, there are strategies to prevent impulse buying; you don't have to be tricked, cajoled, or sweet-talked into buying anything you do not want or need.

With some preplanning and a good mental attitude, you can match wits against the

marketing geniuses. You'll stay on your weight loss program and also save money

in grocery bills each week. (Buy yourself some new clothes with the money you save!)

Here's how to plan your shopping:

First, never take children with you to the store, unless you absolutely have to. A child can be a burden to carry or push around the supermarket, and will likely distract you from the task of buying only what you need. Also, children tend to beg for potentially diet wrecking things, such as candy and snack foods.

The cost of a baby sitter can often be less than the extra amount of groceries you might buy if the child influences you. The reality is, children are great at manipulation; they're adept at influencing you to buy those "munchies" that you simply do not need.

Second, always prepare a grocery list and stick to it. If you've planned your next week's meals (and you should), make a list of exactly what you need for those meals. Do not put anything extra on that list, except for personal health products.

Stick to the list. You'll find that just having a list will keep you from picking up things that you don't need, such as potato chips and cookies.

Look for bargains and coupons, but do not buy problem foods just because they are on sale. Imagine how much money you save by not buying the problem foods at all!

Third, never go grocery shopping when you're hungry. I am sure you have heard that before and that statement is true. Several researchers concluded that when people spend more money when they buy food while they are hungry. The same research shows that shopping on a full stomach results in fewer purchases and less impulse buying.

Try this for yourself the next two times you buy groceries; go once right after a meal, and once when you're hungry. Compare the receipts and you will see all the impulse items you bought while hungry.

When possible, buy foods that require some preparation. That doesn't mean you will be slaving over the stove, though. On the maintenance phase of the diet, you're allowed to eat frozen entrees and all kinds of brand-name foods. But for the upcoming slimming phase, stick to the basics and avoid items like frozen pizzas, etc.

When shopping, check off each item on your list as you select it. Remember, stick to your

list, unless you have to add something necessary. If that is the case, write it down on the list first. Remember, add only necessities, not chips and candy bars.

Fourth, read labels. In fact, become a label reader for the rest of your life. Know what you're eating.

A lot of food packages say one thing on the outside advertising label, and a totally different thing on the list of ingredients. The real story is in the fine print on the list of ingredients; remember to always read the fine print.

Many supposed "diet" or "low calorie" foods are actually neither, and sometimes may contain even more calories (or fat) per serving than their "regular" counterparts. Always read the label to be aware of what you are consuming.

Also, do not be fooled by advertising tricks, which most companies use. For example, the label may list a nominal amount of "calories per serving size", but when you look closer, you see that the serving size is one teaspoon.

Is that a realistic serving size for that particular food? Is it realistic at all?

Be forewarned! Smart shoppers are informed shoppers, who are able to lose weight because they know what they're buying at the grocery store.

The term "low fat" may or may not be good, because the item might contain little fat but lots of sugar. A classic example is flavored yogurt; the label on a strawberry yogurt reads "low fat," but it tells you nothing about the large amount of sugar present in the strawberry preserves used to flavor the yogurt.

Salad dressings are another trap. Many so-called "diet dressings" are lower in calories than their "non-diet" counterparts, but are still relatively dense in calories compared to true diet dressings. My best advice here is to read labels carefully and compare dressings by their calories per tablespoon.

If you find a product with fructose added, be sure it's fructose-90, or a 90% fructose syrup. A few of the soft drink, ketchup, and confection companies are using a less desirable 55% fructose syrup. For purposes of your weight loss program, that is unacceptable.

Also, so-called "sugar free" confections, sweetened with sorbitol and mannitol, must be counted in your diet as calorie-containing foods. Do not mistakenly assume that you can eat these foods without calculating them into your daily intake. For every 10 grams of sorbitol or mannitol you eat, you must deduct one fruit portion from your daily meal plan. (More on portions in the food exchange part of the program).

Make a special effort to avoid ice cream, sherbet, and even ice milk. Be patient; you will be able to eat those, in moderation, when you start the maintenance part of your program. For now, those foods are forbidden. During the slimming phase of this program, you must avoid many dairy products. You will reintegrate many of them back into your diet during maintenance; but you must follow the dairy exchange lists very carefully during the slimming phase.

Be cautious with frozen yogurt, juice pops, gelatin, frozen pudding, and other similar items. They often claim to be made with juices and other natural substances. Guess what most juices contain, and what natural substance they're referring to? You are correct! The answer is sugar.

WHAT TO DO WHEN YOU GET HOME

Put all your purchases away immediately. Do not sample anything; do not snack or nibble. If you live alone, freeze your bread and thaw only enough for a day at a time. Check your menu plans and arrange for easy access only to the permissible foods; avoid contact with things you're not allowed to eat.

Tell other family members that they're not allowed to bring problem foods into the house without first asking you. If you think you can handle having ice cream in the house, then give your permission. If you can't, then put your foot down. Tell the family member that when you reach the maintenance phase, you'll allow them to bring ice cream (or whatever) into the house; but not now.

Be polite, but firm.

MEASURING FOOD

To follow the slimming phase of the program, you're going to have to measure your food. Don't worry, after a while, you will be an expert in what amount of carrots measures to a half-cup or how much beef weighs two ounces.

To start, you need to be familiar with the correct food quantities, whether the amount per portion is given in fluid ounces, ounces of weight, dimensions in inches, or other units. Many people are still confused about what constitutes a cup or an ounce, and rely on their own unsure judgment to help with the measurement. Using proper measurement technique is always better, especially in the initial stages of the program.

Some food-measuring items you will need include several measuring cups; a set of plastic or metal teaspoon and tablespoon measuring spoons; a ruler; and a food scale, preferably with a dish attachment, for convenience. Do not waste money on expensive food scales; an inexpensive one will work just fine.

Practice measuring things. Fill up a glass with a cup of water; see how much of the glass is filled. Put beans or rice on your plate in half-cup and cup sizes; see how much of the plate is covered by the rice or beans. After some practice, you'll be a pro, and eventually you won't have to measure anything (except for ingredients of recipes).

When using salad dressings, be sure to measure carefully. Remember, some salad dressings are almost pure fat, and you are not allowed too much fat on the slimming phase of the program. The soup ladles used in some restaurants to measure their 100 calories/ounce dressing or their 60 calories/ounce "diet dressing" are too generous. You could end up putting 500 or more calories per ladle of dressing on your salad.

FOOD PREPARATION

Your biggest enemy is excess fat in the diet. Fat is the most concentrated of all nutrients and must be dealt with by changing the way foods are cooked.

Most people use too much butter, lard, cream, margarine, cream cheese, and oils in their cooking. Instead of using rich, creamy sauces and gravies, use the natural juices of the foods and avoid smothering the flavors in too many spices and condiments.

Preparation of beef, chicken, and fish stock for soups is a relatively simple procedure; most basic cookbooks include instructions for stock preparation. The majority of the fats present are removed by refrigerating the stock and, after the liquid is sufficiently cooled, getting rid of the upper layer of solidified fat.

Then, you will have stocks available for delicious soups, "dieter's gravies," and other flavor enhancers that increase the taste pleasure of a meal, without adding many calories.

The cooking techniques mentioned here are by no means the only ways to prepare food, but use them as a basic guide for the busy slimmer.

BOILING

I recommend boiling vegetables in an open pan with lots of water. Start off by bringing the water to a boil, add minimal salt, and carefully place the vegetables into the water. Bring the water back to a boil and leave the top off the saucepan. Cook for the recommended amount of time, then drain in a colander. Serve as soon as possible.

Many cooks believe that a small amount of water in a covered pan is better, but I usually use the "Cordon Bleu" method, with an open pan and lots of boiling water.

Parboiling is a variant of boiling. Dense vegetables, such as root vegetables, are partially boiled first, and then fried, without grease or fats. Parboiling is fine, provided the frying is done on a non-stick cooking surface or a regular pan, sprayed with PAM. For a relatively fat-free, parboiled dish, try Pommes Frites a la Cooper (refer to Appendix A for the recipe).

When using mushrooms or tomatoes as a vegetable that will accompany an entrée, do not boil or parboil either one. That rule does not apply when cooking soups or sauces. Most meats, fish, seafood, and poultry can be boiled or parboiled; remove the fat and use the rich stocks and juices as flavor enhancers.

STEAMING

Certain vegetables, including beets, kohlrabi, yams, sweet potatoes, tomatoes, and "greens", such as collards or turnip greens, should usually not be steamed. The remainder of the vegetables listed in this book are generally suitable for full cooking by steaming, or partial cooking (five minutes or less) on a stovetop or counter steamer.

Steaming for five minutes or less will preserve the vitamins and minerals and will not break down the cellulose structure of a vegetable. When that cellulose structure is broken down, usually by overcooking, the caloric content of the vegetable rises. The cellulose structure allows your body to get the nutrients in a vegetable, without absorbing all the calories; however, when vegetables are cooked too long, the cellulose breaks down, and you absorb more of the calories.

The exchange lists define "free vegetables," which are vegetables you can eat whenever you want, in whatever amount you want, as long as they are not fully cooked. Once the vegetable is cooked for five minutes or longer, it is no longer considered a "free vegetable" and must be accounted for in your daily intake.

In addition to vegetables, almost any meat, poultry, or fish dish can be prepared by steaming; the trick is to steam it long enough, particularly poultry, to properly cook it. You can find recommended steaming times for various foods in most good cookbooks or via the internet.

FRYING

Remember that fat is a slimmer's enemy and frying almost always means fat. So, first, try to think of another way to prepare the food that you're thinking about frying. Hide that frying pan, because I seldom want you to use it.

If you must fry, use about one-tenth of what you think you need when you measure out cooking oils or fats. If possible, use none at all! Non-stick pan sprays are excellent aids that permit you to cook without burning foods and without extra, unwanted calories.

Instead of deep-frying, try parboiling or grilling. When properly used, wok cooking is an acceptable variant. A carbon steel wok with a minimum amount of oil at the bottom is often useful. Stir-frying is an art and takes practice, but it produces a smaller amount of extra fat calories to burden the slimmer. Read directions carefully before using one of those utensils.

BAKING

This is another one of my favorite methods of cooking; fruits and vegetables retain their flavor and get very few fat calories. With the use of a dripping pan, meats and other protein foods will have a much lower fat content per ounce because the space between the bottom edge of the meat and the drip pan will eliminate the unwanted fat from submerging the meat.

COOKING WITH WINE

There's nothing wrong with using wine as a flavor enhancer, provided that the alcohol can evaporate during the cooking process. Avoid sauces that are swimming in wine and have their alcohol content unaltered.

GRILLING

I use either a charcoal or gas-fired grill when I cook certain cuts of meat, poultry, and fish. Also, if you can get mesquite wood, it is great for grilling, and it lends a unique flavor to your food.

The meat dishes produced by grilling are quite delicious and have a far lower fat content because of the loss of fatty drippings that fall into the coals or the fire. The hot coals consume the fatty drippings and the smoke comes back up to permeate the meat, producing another unique flavor.

Wrap vegetables in foil or other protective coating (com husks, etc.), prior to grilling them over coals. Potatoes and sweet corn are excellent for grilling, but you should try your own favorites to see how they do.

In summary, when preparing your meals, use as little fat as possible and preserve the natural flavors of the food, instead of smothering it with fatty, high-calorie sauces and gravies.

CHAPTER FIVE

VITAMINS AND MINERALS

"Let food be thy medicine, thy medicine shall be thy food." - Hippocrates

The previous chapter detailed grocery shopping and food preparation. Now, it is time to learn about vitamins, minerals, and antioxidants because understanding their function is instrumental to this program and your weight loss.

WHAT ARE VITAMINS AND MINERALS AND WHY ARE THEY SO IMPORTANT?

Vitamins and minerals are a frequently misunderstood group of substances. They are organic and inorganic nutrients that help our bodies with digestion, absorption, and metabolic processes. In brief, vitamins and minerals act as catalysts in the hundreds of different chemical reactions that constantly take place in the body. Our bodies only need them in small amounts, but they are essential to life.

To understand how vitamins work, we first have to familiarize ourselves with the different classes of vitamins. Vitamins can be broken down into two categories: fat-soluble and water-soluble. Fat-soluble vitamins are stored in fats and fatty tissues of our bodies. We can survive long periods of time without consuming them; ingesting too many fat-soluble vitamins can cause toxicity. Conversely, our bodies do not store large amounts of water-soluble vitamins. Those get excreted into the urine daily.

DO I NEED TO CONSUME VITAMIN/MINERAL SUPPLEMENTS?

Throughout time, vitamins and minerals have been damned for being dangerous and later praised for curing all illnesses. Most nutritionists agree if proper foods are consumed in correct quantities, daily, there is no real need to take vitamin supplements. The majority of the population does not need to take a daily multivitamin. Doctors typically prescribe multivitamins for people with certain medical conditions; those, who recently underwent surgery; those with limited access to nutritious foods; or those with certain lifestyle habits or diets. For example, if you are on an extremely low-fat diet or have fat malabsorption syndromes, consuming a daily multivitamin would be recommended.

Doctors often prescribe a Vitamin D supplement to older people and people with little exposure to sunlight. Folate-rich foods or folic acid supplements reduce the risk of certain birth defects and are prescribed to women of childbearing age. Iron supplements are recommended for pregnant women. Generally, consuming supplements short-term or for a specific purpose is reasonable. But, remember, that food contains many nutrients and other substances that promote general health, so consuming supplements does not substitute for proper food choices.

During the slimming phase of this program, you have to decrease your food intake, which decreases your nutrient intake. As a result, consuming a vitamin and mineral supplement will be helpful because it ensures your body is still getting all the appropriate nutrients. Once you transition to the maintenance portion of the program, you will no longer need additional vitamins and minerals, and should stop consuming the supplement.

SAFETY OF VITAMINS AND MINERALS

The Safety of Supplements, as enacted by the Dietary Supplement Health and Education Act (DSHEA) of 1994, enables consumers to make informed choices about dietary supplements. Prior to marketing, those products are not tested or approved by the FDA, so buyers have to diligently research which vitamins and minerals have good bioavailability. Bioavailability measures how well the nutrient is absorbed based on the various sources it comes from; the greater the bioavailability, the more nutrients are absorbed into the body. Everyone's goal is to absorb the most nutrients, while consuming the least amount of supplements.

Another source of information is the packaging for the supplements. The packaging must provide nutrient information and cannot advertise false health claims; for example, that the supplement is used in diagnosing or treating certain illnesses. The packaging can include the following information: roles of the nutrient; how the compound performs its function; and how consuming the compound is associated with general wellbeing.

WHAT IS AN APPROPRIATE AMOUNT OF VITAMINS FOR DAILY CONSUMPTION?

The federal government established the officially recommended daily amounts of any vitamin or mineral. The minimum daily requirements, or a little more than the minimum, are enough; stay away from the very high potency vitamins and minerals.

I have my own formula that has served my patients well for years. Where the minimum requirement has been established, my formula exceeds the minimum, but not in such high amounts as to pose a health risk. Where there is no set requirement, the adequate amount is estimated by nutritionists and biochemists.

THE DOCTORS' CLINIC-30 FORMULA:

Vitamin B1 (Thiamine)	5 mg
Vitamin B2 (Riboflavin)	5 mg
Vitamin B3 (Niacinamide)	30 mg
Vitamin B5 (as D-Calcium Pantothenate)	10 mg
Vitamin B6 (as Pyridoxine HCL)	2 mg
Vitamin B7 (Biotin)	200 mcg
Vitamin B12 (as Methylcobalamin)	40 mcg
Vitamin C (as Ascorbic Acid)	100 mg
Vitamin D3 (from Lanolin)	400 IU
Zinc (as Zn Amino Acid Chelate 50% and Zinc Picolinate 50% "soy free")	15mg

We have taken the above-formula and created a dietary supplement, consisting of one capsule. The capsules are vegetarian, and in addition to all the vitamins in the Doctors' Clinic-30 Formula, other ingredients include vegetable cellulose (capsule), microcrystalline cellulose, and vegetable leucine. The supplements are now available for purchase. (Refer to Appendix B for further details and purchasing information).

The best time to consume your daily vitamins is during the largest meal of the day; not before or after the meal, but right in the middle of the meal. That is because the fillers and coatings of the supplement capsule can upset your stomach. If your stomach is irritated or upset, take an antacid.

BREAKDOWN OF VITAMINS

FAT-SOLUBLE VITAMINS - A, D, E, AND K

VITAMIN A

ROLES:

- Assists with vision and reproduction
- Protects immune system
- Maintains body's lining and skin (epithelial tissue)
- Promotes bone growth, body growth, and normal cell development

Vitamin A comes in three active forms. The first form is called Retinol; it is stored in our liver, and helps with the conversion of the other active forms of Vitamin A - Retinal and Retinoic Acid. Those help maintain a healthy cornea and function in vision, via light perception, at the retina level.

SOURCES OF VITAMIN A:

- Plants: Mango, cooked carrots, cooked sweet potato, cooked spinach, and apricots.
- Animals: Fortified milk, beef liver, eggs, cheese, and carotenoids.

Below is a list of some Vitamin A pre-cursors, which are found in plants.

- Alpha-Carotene, beta-Carotene, and Beta-Cryptoxanthin can all be converted to retinol and stored in our livers.
- Lycopene (most active form is found in cooked tomato products and protects against prostate and digestive tract cancers), Lutein, and Zeaxanthin do not have Vitamin A activity, but are powerful antioxidants.
- Carotenoids, contained in bright orange colored foods and dark leafy vegetables, are very effective anti-oxidants.

The following formula provides a conversion factor of the different forms of Vitamin A. It is helpful when looking at food labels and supplements in health food stores. Values may vary slightly, depending on the source.

1 microgram (μg) of Retinol = 12 μg of beta-Carotene or 24 μg of other Carotenoids, which can be converted to Retinol and stored in the body.

VITAMIN D

ROLES:

- Maintains calcium and phosphorus levels in the blood, which leads to bone growth and integrity
- Functions as a hormone
- Plays a role in brain, pancreas, skin, reproductive organs, and some cancer cells

Vitamin D (Cholecalciferol) is different than most other vitamins because the body can make it with the help of ultra violet rays from the sun. If a person receives enough sunlight daily, Vitamin D is not an essential nutrient to consume.

SOURCES OF VITAMIN D:

- Plants: Fortified breakfast cereals
- Animals: Fatty (oily) fish: sardines, tuna, and salmon; fortified milk (10 μg/quart in USA)
- Other: Production from sunlight

ADDITIONAL INFORMATION ON VITAMIN D:

Research conducted in recent years has linked Vitamin D deficiency to a myriad of diseases including tuberculosis, psoriasis, multiple sclerosis, inflammatory bowel disease, type-1 diabetes, high blood pressure, heart failure, muscle myopathy, and cancer. Therefore, scientists are calling on the government to increase the recommended daily intake (RDI) of Vitamin D to 2000 International Units (IU). These scientists believe if the occurrence of Vitamin D deficiency was decreased, the incidences of many of those diseases could be reduced by 20-50% or more.

VITAMIN E

ROLES:

- Defends against oxidative damage because of its antioxidant properties
- Protects polyunsaturated fatty acids, and other vulnerable components of the cells and their membranes, from destruction
- Defends against heart disease
- Protects all the cell's lipids and related compounds
- Helps normal nerve development
- Improves immunity by protecting white blood cells

Vitamin E (Tocopherol) has four different Tocopherol compounds; alpha, beta, gamma, and delta. Alpha-Tocopherol is the most active compound.

SOURCES OF VITAMIN E

- Plants: Safflower oil, canola oil, corn oil, wheat germ, mayonnaise, soybeans, and sunflower seeds

ADDITIONAL INFORMATION ON VITAMIN E:

A recent meta-analysis study showed that toxicity occurs in people who take mega-doses of Vitamin E supplements.

VITAMIN K

ROLES:

- Needed in the synthesis of blood-clotting proteins
- Helps with bone formation

Vitamin K has different active forms - Phylloquinone (main dietary source), Menaquinone-7 (in animal products), and Menadiones (synthetic form found in supplements).

SOURCES OF VITAMIN K

- Plants: Cauliflower, cabbage, spinach, lettuce, and garbanzo beans (chickpeas)
- Animals: Beef liver, milk, and eggs

WATER-SOLUBLE VITAMINS – B VITAMINS AND VITAMIN C

Water-soluble vitamins mainly include the B Vitamins and Vitamin C. Cooking and washing can leak these vitamins out of foods; poor storage or light exposure can cause destruction. Unlike with fat-soluble vitamins, the body does not store large amounts of water-soluble vitamins. Toxicity is not an issue because the body can absorb these vitamins easily and excretes them in via urine.

B Vitamins - roles in metabolism help release energy from carbs, fats, and proteins, which then supply energy to the body.

Vitamin B deficiency symptoms include lack of energy, nausea, exhaustion, irritability, depression forgetfulness, loss of appetite, weight loss, muscle pain, impaired immune response, no control of limbs, abnormal heart action, and severe skin problems.

THIAMINE (VITAMIN B1)

ROLES:

- Supports normal appetite and nervous system function
- Easily destroyed by heat and over-exposure to alkaline solutions (baking soda)

Thiamine is part of a coenzyme used in energy metabolism.

SOURCES OF THIAMINE

- Plants: whole grains, legumes, and nuts
- Animals: pork, ham, bacon, and liver

ADDITIONAL INFORMATION ON THIAMINE

- Thiamin Deficiency Symptoms: Beri Beri (wet & dry - thiamine deficiency disease.
  - o Wet: edema, enlarged heart, heart failure, and abnormal heart rhythm.
- Dry: degeneration, wasting, weakness, pain, low morale, difficulty walking, loss of reflexes, mental confusion, and paralysis.
- Thiamine deficiency in alcohol abusers is caused by diminished absorption, excess excretion in urine, and poorer intake of foods containing the vitamin.

- Deficiency leads to a condition called Wernicke-Korsakoff Syndrome, which is characterized by mental confusion, disorientation, memory loss, jerky eye movements, and a staggering gait.

RIBOFLAVIN (VITAMIN B2)

ROLES:

- Helps to support normal vision
- Keeps skin healthy

Riboflavin is a coenzyme used in energy metabolism. The name comes from the Latin word for yellow (Flavin). Small amounts can be stored in the liver, but most excess is excreted in the urine. Excess excretion causes bright yellow urine.

SOURCES OF RIBOFLAVIN

- Plants: leafy greens, whole grain, and enriched breads and cereals
- Animals: milk, yogurt, cottage cheese, and meat

NIACIN (VITAMIN B3)

ROLES:

- Supports health of skin, nervous system, and digestive system
- Functions in energy metabolism

NIACIN SOURCES

- Plants: whole grain and enriched breads, nuts, and all foods containing protein
- Animals: milk, eggs, meat, poultry, and fish

PYRIDOXINE (VITAMIN B6)

ROLES:

- Helps the body use amino acids to make protein and hormones
- Builds new tissues

- Fights infections
- Serves as fuel

Pyridoxine is part of a coenzyme used in amino acid and fatty acid metabolism. It helps convert Tryptophan (the compound in turkey that makes you sleepy) to Niacin, which helps make red blood cells. This vitamin is stored in the muscle, but excess is excreted in the urine.

PYRIDOXINE SOURCES

- Plants: green, leafy vegetables, legumes, fruits, and whole grains
- Animals: meat, fish, poultry, and shellfish

FOLATE (FOLIC ACID)

ROLES:

- Needed for the formation of new cells in the body
- Lowers a woman's risk for cervical cancer
- Decreases the risk of neural tube defects (spina bifida) in women of childbearing age, who consume 400 µg of dietary or synthetic folate, daily.

In some countries, doctors recommend that all women of childbearing age take Folate supplements to avoid birth defects.

FOLATE SOURCES

- Plants: enriched breads, cereal, pasta, grains, green leafy vegetables, legumes, and seeds
- Animals: liver, eggs, and other meat products

CYANOCOBALAMIN (VITAMIN B-12)

ROLES:

- Needed for the formation of new cells in the body
- Helps maintain nerve cells

Cyanocobalamin is similar to Folate; both help cells, like red blood cells and cells that line the digestive tract, multiply.

- Animals: meat, fish, poultry, cheese, and eggs

Vegans usually need supplements, although bacterial contamination of seaweed and other plant foods can be a source.

PANTOTHENIC ACID

Pantothenic acid is part of coenzyme A that - used in energy metabolism. It is also part of the acyl carrier protein that attaches to fatty acids and shuttles them through the pathway designed to increase their chain length, is essential for the metabolism of all macronutrients including alcohol.

PANTOTHENIC ACID SOURCES

Pantothenic is widespread in foods. The vitamin's name comes from the classical Greek word 'pantothen,' which means from every side. In other words, it is found in many foods including milk, meat, liver, peanuts, eggs, yeast, mushrooms, broccoli, etc.

BIOTIN

Biotin is a cofactor for several enzymes used in energy metabolism, fat synthesis, amino acid metabolism, and sugar storage in the liver.

BIOTIN SOURCES

Biotin is widespread in foods. Liver is a rich source. Only few foods have been analyzed for biotin content. Egg white is a very good source, but avudin, a protein found in raw egg white, binds to biotin and prevents absorption. Therefore, eating raw eggs can lead to biotin deficiency and can also cause to salmonella poisoning. Some intestinal bacteria can synthesize biotin.

ASCORBIC ACID (VITAMIN C)

Ascorbic Acid, -vitamin C, Functions as an antioxidant, in collagen and thyroxine (thyroid hormone) synthesis, and in amino acid metabolism. Collagen -strengthens blood vessel walls and, forms scar tissue and; matrix for bone metabolism strengthens resistance to infection and helps in absorption of iron; Vitamin C deficiency will result in a condition called scurvy, which can cause a host of medical problems if not corrected.

ASCORBIC ACID SOURCES:

- Animal: animals contain extremely low amounts, and one cannot prevent deficiency if other food sources are not included in the diet. Human milk contains small amounts to prevent deficiency in infants up to a maximum of 6 months of age.
- Plants: all fruits and vegetables, and fortified foods

VITAMIN C AND THE COMMON COLD:

No study to date has conclusively proved that vitamin C can prevent colds or reduce their severity.

Researchers have lately concluded that vitamin C in amounts up to 1 gm/day may shorten duration of cold by ~ 1 day and reduces severity of symptoms by ~23%.

- Effect may be greater in children than adults.
- In adults, 2 or more g/day may be required to -produce an effect.

WHY DOES IT WORK?

Vitamin C's antioxidant or other activities may boost body's immunity or somehow improve the body's defenses. May act as a weak antihistamine by deactivating histamine

WARNING!

500mg vitamin C it may destroy vitamin B12 if taken within one hour of each other.

MINERALS

CALCIUM

How Much Ca^{2+} Do I Need?

Ca^{2+} absorption varies with age, vitamin D status, Ca^{2+} in diet, and Ca^{2+} binders in foods.

Recommended intakes are high for young and old people.

Obtaining enough Ca^{2+} during young years ensures peak bone mass.

Obtaining enough Ca^{2+} later in life helps minimize bone losses throughout life.

SOURCES OF CALCIUM:

- Animal cheese, milk, and sardines and other fish with bones
- Plant: broccoli, turnip greens, spinach, tofu, and black-eyed peas

PHOSPHORUS

Phosphorous is the second most abundant mineral in the body after calcium. Roughly -85% of phosphorus is found in combination with Ca2+ in bones and teeth. The remaining 15% is distributed throughout the body. Functions of phosphorous include maintaining acid-base balance of cellular fluid, and it, - is essential for growth and renewal of tissues. In metabolism, phosphorus compounds carry, store, and release energy. Phosphorus compounds also assist enzymes and vitamins in extracting energy from nutrients. Luckily, amount of daily phosphorus needed is easily met by almost any diet and deficiencies are unknown.

SOURCES OF PHOSPHOROUS:

Proteins from Animal sources are best. These include dairy products, eggs, meat, fish, and poultry

MAGNESIUM

Only about 30g of magnesium is present in a 130-pound body. Over half of that amount is found in the bones. Another portion is in the muscles, heart, liver, and other soft tissues. Only 1% is in body fluids. If levels are too low, the supply of magnesium in the bones may be used and the kidneys can act to conserve magnesium. Magnesium assists in the operation of more than 300 enzymes. It is needed for the release and the use of energy from energy-yielding nutrients. It directly affects metabolism of potassium, Calcium, and vitamin D. It works with Calcium in contraction/relaxation of muscles. It promotes resistance to tooth decay by keeping calcium in tooth enamel. Magnesium deficiency can occur in many situations including poor intake, vomiting, diarrhea, alcoholism, certain diuretics or protein malnutrition. Magnesium deficiency may be related to heart disease, heart attack, and high blood pressure. Overt deficiency is rare in normal, healthy people.

Magnesium toxicity is often reported in older people who abuse magnesium-containing laxatives, antacids, and other medications.

The consequences of toxicity are diarrhea, acid-base imbalance, kidney impairment, lack of coordination, confusion, coma, and in extreme cases death from heart failure

SOURCES OF MAGNESIUM:

- Animal: seafood, chocolate, and yogurt
- Plant: black beans, black-eyed peas, avocado, spinach and other dark green vegetables, bran, cereals, soy milk and nuts

SODIUM

Sodium is the positive ion in sodium chloride (table salt). Sodium helps maintain acid-base balance and is essential to muscle contraction and nerve transmission. No known human diet lacks sodium. Excess of sodium will be excreted as soon as enough water is drunk to carry salt out of body. Recommended Daily Value (RDA) for sodium is 1,500 mg or less, which is equal to 3.8 g of table salt. The World Health Organization emphasizes moderation as its key concern about sodium. Cultures vary in their use of salt. The average U.S. man consumes 3,300 mg of sodium, or more than 8 g of salt, a day. Asians may consume the equivalent of approximately --30-40 g per day of salt. People with salt sensitivity usually include those with kidney disease, those of African descent, those with family history of high blood pressure, and anyone greater than > 50 years of age. Those with salt sensitivity may respond to lowered salt intake, while others may not. Cutting down on sodium may cause stroke in older people without clinical hypertension. Causes increased calcium excretion from bones. May stress a weakened heart or aggravate kidney problems. Cut down on processed foods, and, - fast foods. Control the salt shaker.

POTASSIUM

Potassium is the principle positively charged ion inside body cells. It-plays a major role in maintaining fluid and electrolyte balance and cell integrity. It is critical in maintaining heart contractions. When brain cells lose potassium, the person loses the ability to notice the need for water, which can be very dangerous.

SOURCES OF POTASSIUM:

- Animal: fish and milk
- Plant: bananas, baked potato, lima beans, and melon

CHLORIDE

Chloride is the major negative ion in the body. It accompanies sodium in fluids outside the cells, and accompanies potassium in fluids inside the cells. It also helps maintain crucial fluid balance in our body, which is important considering two-thirds of our body, is water. Chloride - also helps maintain the strong acidity of the stomach in the form of hydrochloric acid (HCl). This strong acid helps digest food properly.

FOOD SOURCES:

- Salt.

SULFUR

Sulfur is not used by itself as a nutrient. It is present in essential nutrients (thiamine and all proteins). It helps proteins assume functional shape such as in: skin, hair, and nails. There is no recommended intake and deficiencies are unknown.

IODINE

Iodine is critical but only needed by the body in a very small amount. Iodine is part of the thyroid hormone,-thyroxine, - which is responsible for metabolic rate. If iodine concentration is low, cells of the thyroid gland enlarge trying to trap as much iodine as possible. This can become a visible lump on the neck, which is called goiter. Cretinism is iodine deficiency in infants, and leads to mental and physical retardation.

Iodine in food varies – depends on the soil. Iodine is plentiful in the ocean, so seafood is a dependable source. In central parts of U.S. where soil is iodine-poor, iodized salt and food from iodine rich areas has wiped out iodine deficiency. Excessive iodine intake can lead to an - enlarged thyroid gland that resembles goiter. Excess iodine in U.S. is due to our western diet of fast food and additives to milk and bakery products.

IRON

Iron is contained in every living cell and it has a major role to play in the human body. In the simplest terms, it helps carry oxygen to tissues and hold in the muscle. It also needed to make new cells, amino acids, hormones, and neurotransmitters

Iron deficiency is the most common nutrient deficiency in the world. Affects approximately - 40% of world's population, with highest prevalence in developing countries; the population that is especially vulnerable include older infants, young children, and pregnant women.

WHAT CAUSES IRON DEFICIENCY?

- Malnutrition
- Over consumption of foods rich in fat and sugar and poor in nutrients
- Blood losses, - approximately -80% of iron is in the blood.
- Women before the menopause need 1½ times as much iron as men due to menstrual losses.

Iron deficiency anemia – a form of anemia caused by iron deficiency. In anemia, you cannot deliver oxygen to the body cells as efficiently. Therefore, some of the symptoms you might experience are tiredness, apathy, and tendency to feel cold. These symptoms disappear when iron intake improves either from dietary sources or supplements.

Iron is toxic in large amounts. Iron overload can be caused by overconsumption and by a hereditary defect that causes the intestine to helplessly absorb excess iron. Tissue damage occurs especially in iron-storing organs (liver), and infections are likely because bacteria thrive on iron-rich blood. Excess iron has been linked to heart disease and colon cancer.

RECOMMENDATIONS FOR IRON:

Best to rely on iron from foods because iron from supplements is much less absorbed

RDA for men	10 mg/day
RDA for women age 19-50	15 mg/day
RDA for women age 51 and up	10 mg/day

SOURCES OF IRON:

- Animal (Heme iron): meat, poultry, fish, clams, and beefsteak
- Plant: spinach, enriched cereal, navy beans, and tofu

Heme iron is much more readily absorbed than nonheme iron. Meat, fish, and poultry contain a factor - MFP factor - that promotes absorption of heme iron.

Vitamin C also promotes iron absorption. Factors that impair iron absorption include tea, coffee, calcium and phosphorus in milk, and phytates that accompany fiber in whole grain cereals.

ZINC

Zinc is stored in a very small quantity in the body but works with proteins in every organ.

Zinc helps -catalyze more than fifty reactions in our body. It also helps make parts of the cells' genetic material. It helps the pancreas with its digestive functions, and helps metabolize protein, fat, and carbohydrate.

Zinc also does the following: liberates vitamin A from storage in the liver; disposes of damaging free radicals (part of the antioxidant process); affects behavior and learning; and assists in immune function. It is essential to wound healing, fetal development, taste perception, sperm production, and growth and development in children. It is needed to produce active form of vitamin A

Zinc deficiency impairs all of these and other functions including altering digestive function. Therefore zinc deficiency can result in diarrhea, impaired immune response, and can lead to vitamin deficiencies, which can slow down the energy metabolism in the body. There is also a loss of appetite/impaired taste sensitivity that patients may describe and, as well as, decreased wound healing.

Too much Zinc may hamper iron absorption in the body as well as compete with copper for absorption leading to copper deficiency this can lead to several neurological problems. This is more commonly seen in patients that underwent recent gastric bypass surgery and patients who wear dentures as the paste that is applied for the dentures contains zinc and overuse has been reported with copper deficiency.

SOURCES OF ZINC:

- Animal: shellfish, beef and other meats; cheese, poultry, yogurt
- Plant: enriched cereal and legumes

SELENIUM

Selenium plays a role in antioxidant enzyme activity. It protects vulnerable body chemicals from oxidation by preventing formation of free radicals. It also has a, - role in activating thyroid hormones. Anyone who eats a normal diet composed of mostly unprocessed foods need not worry about consuming enough selenium.

Most people in U.S. receive plenty of selenium.
- Deficiency: specific type of heart disease.
- Toxicity: hair loss, diarrhea, nerve abnormalities.

FLUROIDE

Fluoride is not essential to life, but is beneficial in that it helps inhibits dental caries and stabilizes bones.

Too much fluoride can lead to discoloring of teeth. Large doses are toxic. Drinking water is usual source, unless it is not supplemented.

CHROMIUM

Chromium works closely with the hormone insulin (when chromium is lacking, insulin action is impaired). Studies have shown no effect of chromium on weight loss and building of muscle.

Chromium in foods and supplements seems to be relatively nontoxic in amounts of approximately 200 µg/day. Most U.S. adults have low intakes of chromium. Chromium is lost during processing.

Best sources: liver, whole grains, nuts, cheeses, meats, fats, and vegetable oils.

COPPER

Copper helps form hemoglobin and collagen. It assists in reactions leading to the release of energy, and works with proteins to regulate activity of certain genes.

COPPER SOURCES:

- Organ meats, seafood, nuts, seeds, and sometimes water (contamination through copper pipes)

MOLYBDENUM

Molybdenum functions as part of several metal-containing enzymes.

MANGANESE

Manganese works with dozens of different enzymes that facilitate different body processes.

All trace minerals are toxic in excess. Obtain all trace minerals from food, which is not hard to do.

A LITTLE ABOUT ANTIOXIDANTS AND HOW THEY CAN HELP YOU GET HEALTHY AND STAY HEALTHY

The recommendations of the National Institute of Health, the National Cancer Institute, the National Heart and Lung Institute, the American Heart Association, the American Cancer Society and other equally prestigious sources of medical information state,- that the amount of fruits and vegetables in our diet can be increased. The usual figure given is about eight to ten helpings of fresh fruits and vegetables, along with a certain amount of whole grain foods. Only about nine percent of Americans get as many as three. Dozens of experimental studies have shown that with the proper amount of fruits and vegetables, we can neutralize a particularly dangerous group of substances in our bodies called free radicals, which damage our cells and our DNA.

Free radicals are molecules generated by certain oxidative processes in the body, or by contact with a number of toxic substances. Even sunlight is potentially dangerous. Once these free radicals are produced, they circulate throughout the body and do their dirty work. They resemble bees in their ability to "sting" the cell membranes or the inner parts of the cells, including the DNA on the chromosomes of each cell. When the free radicals comes in contact with a cell membrane, the negatively, - charged "stinger" of each free radical molecule will damage the membrane. Enough hits without some sort of repair work and the cell quits functioning or dies. If DNA inside the chromosomes of the cell is damaged, we can do some repair work, but sometimes the DNA is changed by these oxidative hits and the cell can no longer reproduce and renew itself. An even worse thing happens if the cell begins to multiply in an uncontrolled manner and the result is a tumor or an actual malignant cancer.

We all age and we all must eventually die, but if we neutralize these free radicals with natural substances in fruits, vegetables, and grains (antioxidants), we can minimize or reverse damage caused by these substances. There are three ways to get enough antioxidants to protect ourselves.

Eat 8 to 10 helpings of fresh fruits, vegetables and grains a day, preferably only lightly cooked or steamed. Cost is $6.00 to $10.00 a day.

Take the same amount of these healthy foods as in (1), juice them and drink the juices every day. Cost is the same, but there is more mess to clean up, including the juicer.

Take a commercially available, whole food preparation made from 17 different fruits, vegetables, and grains every day. The juice is cold processed and dried at low temperatures, and the entire product, is in individual, easy to swallow doses. Cost of this method is from $1.50 to as low as $1.35 per day. This is less than people spend on a soda and a bag of chips.

Any one of these three methods of getting antioxidants into the body will work. There is no reason we shouldn't live to be over 100 and maintain our energy, sex drive, and other faculties during the entire life span. The only catch is that you have to help your body by cutting out things that stress your body and cause aging.

Obesity itself increases risk of coronary heart disease, high blood pressure, type II diabetes, and various cancers by 300 to 600%. Doesn't eating the type of healthy foods that can provide us with that type of protection?

CHAPTER SIX

A NEW AND SLIMMER YOU

"Take care of your body. It's the only place you have to live." – Jim Rohn

You're almost ready to begin the slimming phase of The Doctors' Clinic-30 Program. You have only one more thing to do: you must set a reasonable goal weight. Now, I told you in an earlier chapter that I don't want you to be a slave to your scale, and I mean it.

I don't even want you to weigh yourself for the first couple weeks of the program, but you have to know when to stop. Beyond that, you have to set a reasonable goal, not some silly goal of weighing what you did in high school.

I highly recommend that you set goals in stages; once you reach one stage, set a second goal, reach it and go on. If you've been overweight a long, long time, don't expect to reach your ideal weight right away. Take things one step at a time; do not expect to lose more than ten pounds a month on this program.

I like the "rule of thumb" method for calculating how much you should weigh. Measure your height in your stocking feet. Women, who are five feet tall, should weigh 100 pounds; however, if you have a large frame, add 10%, and if you have a slight frame, subtract 10%. Thus, the weight range for a five-foot tall woman is 90 to 110 pounds, depending on whether she has a slight, medium, or large frame. For every inch over five feet, add five pounds. Thus, a woman who is five feet and six inches tall, with a medium frame, should weigh about 130 pounds; there is a range of 13 pounds below or above that figure, depending on the size of her bone structure, or frame.

For men, start out with a basic weight of 106 pounds for the first five feet, and add six pounds for every inch over that height. Again, we add or subtract 10% for large or small frames. Thus, a man who is six feet tall should weigh 160 to 196 pounds, depending on his frame.

As you can see, this leaves both men and women with a pretty wide range, which is good. You should be losing weight to improve your health and your quality of life, not to reach some magical and mythical figure that you pull out of the air.

Be reasonable with yourself. You want to look good, but do not expect unrealistic results.

Look at yourself in front of a full-length mirror, without any clothes on. Imagine what you'll look like at your ideal weight. Now, add five or ten pounds; you'd still look pretty good.

Again, be reasonable. You'll know how much to lose and what weight to stop at as you approach your ideal weight. Use the "rule of thumb" method as a guide, not as an absolute.

We will discuss what to do once you reach your weight goal a little later.

AN EASY WAY TO DETERMINE WHAT TO EAT AND HOW MUCH

In our busy and hectic society, no one has time to count calories or grams. Many of you are raising families with two income earners and simply cannot pause your daily schedules to cook different types of special dishes.

The beauty of the exchange system is that it lets you pick and choose what you should eat, based on how many exchanges, or portions, of each food group you're allowed each day.

With some variations, the exchange system has been around for over 40 years.

Basically, you can "exchange" different foods within the same food group as equivalent portions. Each of these different foods in the same category has about the same amount of calories, protein, carbohydrates, and fat.

Because it allows for a "free exchange" of equivalent portions of each food group, it's called the exchange system. Throughout the book, the terms "exchange" and "portion" are used interchangeably because, for purposes of this program, they mean exactly the same thing. When you see a food item and an amount such as ½ cup listed in the following charts, you'll know that amount constitutes one portion or one exchange.

The determination of what makes up a portion or exchange can be a futile exercise in guesswork if you don't measure foods to start. Make sure you have the basic food measuring tools. Remember, after a short while, you'll be able to "eyeball" most foods and figure out their portions;

however, check yourself periodically to make sure you don't start making your portions a little larger than they should be.

Make sure you measure meat, poultry, or fish after they are cooked, not before. An ounce of beef, lamb, pork, liver, chicken, turkey, or veal will usually measure 3 inches by 2 inches by one-eight inch. Again, time and practice will make you experienced enough to judge the size of each type of portion in each category of food. A four-ounce portion will be about the size of a deck of cards.

The beauty of this program is that it allows you to interchange freely within each food group, and allows you to plan your own meals. For example, if you're going to do a lot of physical work during the day, then you want to make sure you have a larger breakfast and lunch, and a moderate or light dinner. You can easily accomplish that by using more of your exchanges during breakfast and lunch, and fewer of them for dinner.

If you want to have a snack, that's easy, too. Just remove a portion from one meal and eat it whenever you like. You can eat up to six meals a day on this plan; always remember to stay within the allotted daily portions for each food group.

I must emphasize one thing — I want you to use all your portions up, every day. Some people want to lose weight fast, and figure they'll eat less than their daily allotment. That is a bad idea, which could lead to serious health problems. Your body needs all the nutrients it will get from this program, and you cannot cut things out. Eat all your portions every day; if you follow this program, you'll lose weight.

The food tables make planning your meals, either for the day or for the week, very easy. You might want to photocopy them and put them up on the cupboard. Keep the food lists handy, for reference; pretty soon, you'll know the amounts of foods and you'll hardly have to refer to them.

Think of these food exchanges or portions as money. When you use them up for the day, they're gone. There is no such thing as a credit card on this plan. When your money's gone that day, it's gone. However, unlike money, you'll get a new allotment of food portions the next day.

Keep in mind that you cannot substitute one category of food for another. For example, if you use all three fruit portions in a day, you cannot substitute a meat or bread portion for a fruit portion. If you use all three fruit portions, then you can't eat any more fruit that day.

There is no easier way to keep track of what you eat. This program has been tried and tested for more than four decades, and it works.

Many of you are wondering whether you can eat a restaurant; the answer is a qualified "yes." You can go out to a regular restaurant and eat, as long as you are mindful of your portions. If you know you're allowed one or two meat portions, one or two bread portions, one vegetable portion, etc., just order accordingly. If the steak comes in an 8-ounce size, and you only have three 1-ounce meat exchanges left, then eat only three ounces, and take the rest home in a doggie bag; order a smaller steak; or give half to your dining partner.

What I'm trying to drive home is that you can eat out; just use a little planning and forethought. However, at least during the slimming part of this program, you should not go to fast-food restaurants. It is no secret that the salt, sugar, and fat contents of most fast food are unbelievable! You cannot consume the fat and sugar, and still lose weight. Be patient. Once on maintenance, you'll occasionally be able to eat at a fast-food restaurant, although you really have to watch the calories in such food.

In the beginning of this program, you should cook most of the food yourself. Do not rely on prepared foods, such as frozen dinners or frozen pizza. Once you reach your desired weight, there are plenty of good frozen entrees, canned soups, and foods that you can eat. In fact, most of them are listed by brand name in the maintenance section of this program. For the slimming phase, it is important that you stay away from such foods. However, if you must eat prepared or canned foods during the slimming phase, look ahead to the maintenance section in the next chapter to get the exchange equivalents for the particular food. Then figure the exchanges into your daily allotment.

You must drink water and other beverages on this program. Water is really good for you; it helps you lose weight, helps your liver and kidneys function properly, and helps your skin to stay healthy during weight loss.

Try to get at least 80 to 90 ounces of fluid a day, and most of that should be water.

You can have up to two caffeine-containing drinks (coffee, tea, sugar-free sodas) a day. Drink coffee and tea without any cream, but artificial sweeteners with no calories may be used as desired.

If you want to use some of your rations of skim milk for your coffee, do so, but be sure to count them. You may have up to 10 envelopes of Equal or Sweet 'n Low daily. You can also have some sugar-free, caffeine-free sodas and other beverages each day. Remember, moderation is key to your weight loss success.

If you aren't used to that much fluid intake, start lower and gradually raise your daily intake amount, until you reach at least 80 to 90 ounces. Mineral water and sugar-free drinks such as Kool-Aid are also permitted. Avoid "punch" drinks like Sunny Delite, Frutopia, Splash, Gatorade, and others with lots of sugar. Most drinks have nutrition labels; if there are more than three calories per eight ounces, avoid the drink entirely.

If you drink milk, (only skim or reconstituted dry milk is currently permitted), you must make sure to account for it; during the sliming phase, avoid two percent and whole milk.

Drinking a lot of fruit juice is discouraged; it is better to eat the fruits themselves. Cranberry juices, and other juices with a high content of corn syrup sweeteners, are particularly bad choices. As always, the best drink of all is water.

Follow the slimming phase of the program until you reach your goal weight, or a weight close to that. Then, you must start the maintenance phase. Remember, losing weight is just part of what you need to do. You have to maintain that weight loss for the rest of your life via behavior change and exercise.

HOW TO HANDLE SNACKING

Snacking is a pattern of life for many of us. Some people eat a proper breakfast, but many of us have a skimpy one, or skip it altogether. When that happens, hunger hits about 10:30 in the morning and you have nothing to reach for, besides a cheese Danish laden with fat and calories.

At night, while glued to the television, millions of people pile on the calories. That's because watching TV is a passive activity, where you don't burn any calories; often times, you don't realize how much you are eating, while sitting in front of the TV.

What are you to do about this? You must break old habits, but you cannot do that unless you replace those old habits with something else. And, if you must snack, then you have to make the right choice about snacking.

What you put into your mouth will affect your life. Think about that for a moment. What kinds of things do you want to put in your mouth? Candy bars? Potato chips? Chocolate sundaes?

You substitute your favorite snacks with things like: thin slices of apples and cheese; sweet fruits or ripe pears cut into small pieces; celery sticks or sauerkraut (if you have the urge for something salty). There are plenty of alternatives that allow you to snack and still eat healthy, lose weight; and maintain your weight loss.

The first thing you have to do is change the way you think about snacks. Snacks don't have to include candy bars, potato chips, and all the rest. Start thinking of snacks as portions of your meal that you set aside for later: fruits and vegetables; wonderful bran muffins; low-calorie soups that are filling; even ice-cold drinks made with fresh fruits and sugar substitutes.

Another thought that might be unusual to some of you is to stop thinking of snacks only as food. Physical and mental activities can be snacks, too — taking a walk when you get the urge to eat; cleaning the basement; making love; watching and listening to the birds in your backyard; reading that novel you've been meaning to read; meditating; or just reflecting on life.

Snacking on junk and calorie-laden foods is an acquired habit, and it can be broken only if you replace it with something else: snacking on the right kinds of food; saving a portion of your meal for later; or replacing the urge to eat with some physical or mental activity.

If snacking at the office is a real problem for you, plan ahead. If you cannot fight them, join them. But join them on your own turf. For example, when somebody passes by and offers you a Danish, or if somebody is making a "run" to the deli, politely refuse and bring out your own snack, one you prepared the night before. Just because everyone else is snacking on 200 to 400 calories, doesn't mean you have to. Enjoy your healthy snack.

What's a good healthy snack for the office? Instead of Danish or doughnuts, bring a homemade oat bran muffin with a thin layer of jelly on top. Not just any jelly, but the kind that is virtually all fruit. It's sold in the stores now. (There are some excellent muffin recipes in Appendix A of this book). That's just one idea; there are plenty of alternatives for you.

What about snacking at night? That is also hard to overcome. Usually you sit in front of the television and watch plenty of commercials for all kinds of food, from potato chips to pizza. And the pizza will be delivered right to your door. How can you resist?

You start by removing all unhealthy snacks from your house. Your family is going to need to cooperate and it might not be easy to get their assistance. But you must be firm, and put your foot down. While you're losing weight, the kids have to give up Oreo cookies if they are one of your problem foods. Be firm on this, or you'll lose the battle before it starts. It's easy to snack on junk food, if you keep it around the house; it's less convenient to climb in the car and drive to the store to buy the junk food.

When you get a snack attack, view the situation. If boredom is causing your hunger, then do something about the boredom; do not feed it! If you're having true hunger, then plan ahead and remove a portion or two from your meal to eat as a snack. If you didn't do that and are experiencing true hunger, then you have a choice to make. You can either eat a healthy snack, or one that will cause weight gain; the decision is solely up to you.

Remember, if you're going to snack, don't eat mounds of food. Begin to cut back and eat foods that aren't calorie-dense like cottage cheese, fruits, or raw vegetables. If you're craving something salty, slice a cucumber, soak it in vinegar for a few minutes, drain it well, and eat it; the craving for salt will be curbed by your healthy snack.

At night, I like cereal with skim milk and sugar substitute. It's as sweet as a sundae. I eat it slowly and chew every mouthful. Snacks, like regular meals, should not be shoveled in. Count what you eat as a snack in your daily portions, the amount you're allowed each day. You can eat up to six meals a day by saving some portions for later, when you might be hungry.

Finally, there are many vegetables you can snack on that are free foods, which means they don't count as a portion or exchange. These vegetables make excellent snacks, too, if eaten in reasonable quantities. You can dip them into salsa, which has virtually no calories; that way you aren't eating chips or a high-fat dip. Alternatively, lightly steamed vegetables make great snacks.

BEWARE OF FOOD CLAIMS

Beware of fat-free chains, especially if the items are loaded with sugar, as they usually are. One particularly guilty company has promoted fat-free cookies and related products, giving the compulsive eater a treacherous false sense of security. One of my patients referred to this type of "fat-free" cookie as the "Antichrist of Diet Foods." Regardless of what you think, you must be careful and be a label reader.

If a "fat-free" food has a great sugary taste, then, if you buy it, you are in trouble as a dieter. Look for ingredients ending in "ose" (glucose, sucrose) or products that have "syrup" (corn syrup solids, etc.) Confections sweetened with grape juice or other fruit juices are probably OK to have, but look at the caloric content of each serving. If you're unsure whether something is allowable on your diet, it is best to avoid that product.

THE BENEFITS OF FRUITS AND VEGETABLES TO YOUR HEALTH

In June of 1997, the New England Journal of Medicine published an article about an experiment, which resembled The Doctors' Clinic-30 Program. Dr. Thomas Vogt, of the Kaiser Permanente Center for Health Research, noted a significant drop in blood pressures of study subjects, within two weeks of starting a diet rich in vegetables and fruits. Dr. Vogt estimated that there would be 125,000 fewer strokes every year, if everyone in the United States experienced a similar drop in their blood pressure.

Many medical studies over the past two decades link consumption of fruits and vegetables to a reduced risk of cataracts, coronary heart disease, heart attacks, stroke, and some cancers. The high level of natural antioxidants from these fresh foods seem to have a protective effect on the cells of the body that are attacked by free radicals. Using the antioxidants in fresh fruits and vegetables, those deadly chemicals can be neutralized, so they are then unable to perform their deadly work.

On September 28, 1996, the British Medical Journal published a 17-year study, which found that people who eat fresh fruit daily have a 32% lower incidence of fatal strokes; a 24% less possibility of a fatal heart attack; and a 21% less chance of fatalities from any cause.

Cancer Epidemiology, Biomarkers and Prevention (September 1996) reported that men who ate fresh fruit every day had a 70% less chance of dying from cancer of the digestive tract, particularly the colon.

THE BASIC SIX FOOD GROUPS

There are six basic food groups in this program, and a seventh group of free foods that can be eaten in moderation without counting them in the total scheme of daily food intake. The basic groups are:

- Breads-cereals-pasta
- Fruits
- Dairy products
- Vegetables
- Meat and protein food group
- Fats
- Free Foods

Now, let's review the amount of portions you can eat from each food group.

All men, and any women over 68 inches tall, are allowed: seven portions from the meat and protein food group; two portions from the vegetable group; two portions from the dairy group; three portions from the fruit group; four portions from the bread-cereal-pasta group; one portion from the fat group; and unlimited portions (in moderation) from the free food group.

Women 68 inches tall or shorter can have five portions from the meat and protein group. The rest of the portions are the same as listed above.

You can mix the portions however you want for breakfast, lunch, and dinner — including snacks.

Here's an example of a daily meal plan for a man:

BREAKFAST

Breads-cereal-pasta	one portion
Fruit	one portion
Dairy	one portion
Meat and protein group	one portion

LUNCH

Breads-cereal-pasta	one portion

Fruit	one portion
Meat and protein group	two portions
Vegetables	one portion
Free foods	as desired

DINNER

Breads-cereal-pasta	one portion
Fruit	one portion
Meat and protein group	three portions
Vegetables	one portion
Dairy	one portion
Fat	one portion
Free foods	as desired

SNACK

Breads-cereal-pasta	one portion
Meat and protein group	one portion

From the example above, you can see how this system you great flexibility in planning your meals easily and effectively. The fact that you can exchange all kinds of foods within food groups makes it even easier. Make your selections from the appropriate lists on the following pages.

BREAD-CEREAL-PASTA FOOD GROUP

You are to eat FOUR portions from this group every day.

These foods are from grains, seeds, or roots of plants. They are not all bread-like in appearance, but for our purposes they are essentially identical in nutritional composition to bread.

Each portion contains about 80 calories, the equivalent of one slice of bread. Where there are added fat calories to be accounted for, they are listed in the right-hand "extra" column. When it says "½ fat," this means that you have to account for an extra half-portion of fat, subtracting it from your daily allowance.

During the weight loss phase of The Doctors' Clinic-30 Program, you have only one daily fat portion to subtract, so you should probably omit these bread-like foods from you diet until you are ready to go to the maintenance program. Sometimes, you won't be able to do that, so I've listed them here to enable you to account for them in your daily allowance.

When you reach your ideal weight, the fat content and the number of calories allowed will be greater.

Some items in the bread group, notably cereals, also contain fruit. We have to account for that. When it says "½ fruit" in the "extra" column, omit a half-portion of fruit from your daily allowance.

If something is not on the list below, then it isn't allowed. That goes for the other food group lists as well. Those items with a higher content of fiber are marked with an asterisk (*) and are preferred over those not marked that way.

BREADS AND BAKED GOODS

Type of Product	Amount per Portion	Extra Portion & Type
Bagel	½ bagel	
Biscuits from mix	1 biscuit	½ fat
Biscuit, buttermilk	1 biscuit	½ fat
Biscuit, flaky	1 biscuit	1 fat
Bread, Hollywood	1 slice	
Bread, rye	1 slice	
Bread, white or French	1 slice	
Bread, whole wheat	1 slice	
Breadsticks, crisp 4"xl/2"	2 sticks (⅔ oz.)	
Bun, hamburger/frankfurter	½ bun (1 oz.)	
Combread	1 piece, 1½" square	1 fat
Croutons, plain	½ cup	
English muffin	½ muffin	
Malsovit bread*	1 slice	
Malsovit Mealwafer*	1 wafer	
Matzo cracker	1 cracker, 6" square	

Type of Product	Amount per Portion	Extra Portion & Type
Melba toast	5 pieces	
Muffin, bran, homemade*	one 2" muffin	1 fat
Muffin, corn, homemade	one 2" muffin	1 fat
Pancakes from mix	2 pancakes, 3" diam.	
Pita bread	½ of 6" pocket	
Popover from mix	½ popover	½ fat
Raisin bread, unfrosted	1 slice	
Rice	½ cup, cooked	
Rice cakes	2 cakes	
Roll, brown & serve	1 roll	½ fat
Roll, butterflake	1 roll	½ fat
Roll, crescent	1 roll	1 fat
Roll, croissant, Sara Lee	1 roll	1 fat
Roll, all others	1 roll 2" diam.	
Rusks	2 rusks	
Spoon bread	2 oz. (¼ cup)	1 fat
Taco/tostada shell	2 shells	1 fat
Tortilla	1 tortilla, 6" diam.	
Waffle	1 waffle, 4" square	

CEREALS AND PASTA

Type of Product	Amount per Portion	Extra Portion
All Bran*	⅓ cup	
Alpha Bits	¾ cup	
Apple Jacks	1 cup	1 fruit
Bran, 100%*	½ cup	

Type of Product	Amount per Portion	Extra Portion
Bran Buds*	⅓ cup	
Bran Chex*	½ cup	
Bran Flakes, 40%*	½ cup	
Buc Wheats	½ cup	
Bulgur (cooked)*	½ cup	
Cap'n Crunch	¾ cup	½ fat
Cheerios	¾ cup	
Cocoa Krispies & Pebbles	¾ cup	1 fruit
Cocoa Puffs	1 cup	1 fruit
Cooked cereals not listed	½ cup	
Com bran*	½ cup	
Com Chex	½ cup	
Com flakes	¾ cup	
Com grits, cooked	½ cup	
Com meal, dry	2½ tablespoons	
Com Total	¾ cup	
Count Chocula	1 cup	1 fruit
Cream of Rice, cooked	½ cup	
Cream of Wheat, cooked	½ cup	
Farina, Cooked	½cup	
Fortified oat flakes*	½ cup	
Frankenberry	1 cup	1 fruit
Fruit loops	1 cup	1 fruit
Frosted Miniwheats	4 biscuits	1 fruit
Fruit & Fibre*	⅔ cup	½ fruit
Grape Nuts	¼ cup = 1½ portions	
Grape Nuts Flakes	⅔ cup	

Type of Product	Amount per Portion	Extra Portion
Grits, cooked	½ cup	
Heartland Natural Cereals	¼ cup of any	1 fat
Honeycomb	½ cup	
Kix	1 cup	
Life, plain & cinnamon	⅔ cup	1 fruit
Luck Charms	1 cup	1 fruit
Macaroni, cooked	½ cup	
Most	½ cup	
Noodles, cooked	½ cup	
Noodles, Chow Mein	¼ cup	
Nutrigrain, all types*	½ cup	
Oats, regular, cooked*	½ cup	
Pasta, all types, cooked	½ cup	1 fruit
Product 19	½ cup	
Puffed rice or wheat	1½ cup	
Raisin bran*	½ cup	
Rice chex	¾ cup	
Rice Krispies, plain	⅔ cup	
Roman Meal, cooked*	½ cup	
Shredded Wheat*	1 large biscuit ½ cup	
Spaghetti, cooked, no sauce	⅓ cup	
Special K	1⅓ cup	1 fruit
Sugar-coated cereals	Not recommended	
Team	⅔ cup	
Total	⅔ cup	
Trix	⅔ cup	
Wheat Chex	½ cup	

Type of Product	Amount per Portion	Extra Portion
Wheat & Raisin Chex	½ cup	1 fruit
Wheatena, cooked	½ cup	
Wheaties	⅔ cup	

STARCHY VEGETABLES AND LEGUMES

Type of Product	Amount per Portion
Beans, dried, cooked*	⅓ cup
Beans, baked without pork*	¼ cup
Com, cooked*	½ cup
Com on cob*	1 piece, 6" long
Hominy, cooked*	½ cup
Lentils, dried, cooked*	⅓ cup
Lima beans, cooked*	½ cup
Parsnips, cooked*	1 small
Peas, dried, cooked*	⅓ cup
Peas, green, cooked*	½ cup
Plantain*	½ cup
Potato, sweet / yam, cooked*	⅓ cup
Potato, white, baked*	1 small, 3 oz.
Potatoes, white, mashed	½ cup
Squash, winter, acorn*	¾ cup
Squash, winter, butternut*	¾ cup

CRACKER AND SNACKS

Type of product	Amount per Portion	Extra Portion & Type
Animal crackers	8 crackers	

Type of product	Amount per Portion	Extra Portion & Type
Graham crackers	3 crackers, 2½" square	
Oyster crackers	24 crackers	
Popcorn, airpopped only*	3 cups	
Pretzels	¾ oz.	
Ritz and similar crackers	crackers	
Rye Krisp	crackers	1 fat
Saltines	small squares	
Triscuits	Crackers	
Uneeda biscuits	4 biscuits	

I'm aware there is a certain amount of fiber in most of the items not marked with an asterisk, but those marked with the asterisk are far better for you in terms of fiber content. Popcorn with ANY amount of oil is forbidden. Microwave and stovetop popcorn is a definite no-no, and so is the popcorn purchased from vendors at theaters and in shopping malls. Use air-popped only, at least until you reach your maintenance program!

FRUITS AND FRUIT-LIKE ITEMS

You are to have THREE portions of fruit per day.

Each item included in the fruit and fruit-like list contains about 15 grams of carbohydrate and around 60 calories for the serving or fruit size listed. For each fruit, I've listed the name of the fruit or food, the size serving that equals one portion, and the number of grams of fiber per portion, if this number is at least 0.5 grams or better. Try to pick fruits with a higher fiber content.

Fruits with a C and/or A in parentheses are good sources of those vitamins.

It's a good idea to get fresh, frozen, or dried fruits when possible. Fruits canned in water or their own juices are permitted in moderation, but are inferior in nutrition to those that have not been through the canning process. The word syrup (even light syrup) means that sugar has been added, and that is not desirable for a person on a calorie-restricted program.

Certain foods mentioned in this and other groups will only be available in the United Kingdom, but are included because this book is published there, too. Other fruits will be found only in certain localities during certain seasons. Their inclusion is also for the sake of thorough coverage of the subject.

The whole fruit is always far superior to the juice, which does not contain the pulp, water-soluble fiber, and bulk of the entire fruit portion. For example, two portions of apple juice can be consumed in just a few seconds, but two apples will take many times longer to eat and will provide more satisfaction to you. Trust me.

NOTE: When no figures are given for the fiber content of a fruit portion listed below, it means that we either don't know this information, or the quantity is below 0.5 grams per portion.

Name of Fruit	Size of Portion	Grams Fiber
Apple, 1 small	2" diameter	1.1
Apple, dried	4 rings	0.7
Apple juice, unsweetened	½ cup	
Applesauce, unsweetened	½ cup	0.7
Apricots, raw (A)	4 medium	0.8
Apricots, dry (A)	7 halves	0.7
Avocados — Not counted as a fruit;	see fat portion list.	
Banana, raw	½ of 9" fruit	
Banana flakes	2 rounded tablespoons	
Bilberries, raw	½ cup	
Blackberries, raw	¾ cup	4.5
Blueberries, raw (A/C)	¾ cup	1.4
Boysenberries, frozen	1 cup, unsw.	3.6
Breadfruit, raw (C)	1/6 small	0.9
Cantaloupe, raw (A/C)	⅓ of 5" melon	0.6
Cantaloupe, chunks (A/C)	1 cup	0.6
Cherries, sweet, raw	12 cherries	
Cherries, canned, waterpack	½ cup	

Name of Fruit	Size of Portion	Grams Fiber
Crenshaw melon	3" wedge	0.5
Currants, all colors, raw	1 cup	2.6
Dates, dried, unglazed	2½ medium	0.5
Date "sugar"	1½ tablespoons	
Elderberries, raw (A/C)	½ cup	5.0
Figs, raw, 2" across	2 figs	1.1
Figs, dried, 2" across	1½	0.7
Fructose, granulated	1 rounded tablespoon	
Fructose syrup	1½ tablespoons	
Fruit cocktail, waterpacked	¾ cup	0.9
Gooseberries, raw, sections	1 cup	2.9
Grapefruit, raw (C)	½ medium	
Grapefruit juice, unsw.(C)	½ cup	
Grapefruit sections (C)	½ cup	
Grapes, small	15 grapes	0.7
Grape juice, unsw.	⅓ cup	
Guava, raw (C)	1 medium	5.0
Haws, scarlet, raw	2½ oz.	1.5
Honeydew melon, raw (C)	1/8 medium melon	
Honeydew melon chunks (C)	1 cup chunks	
Kiwi fruit, raw (C)	1 large kiwi	0.8
Kumquats, raw (A/C)	5 medium	4.0
Lemons, raw (C)	3 medium	0.6
Lemon juice, fresh (C)	1 cup	
Limes, raw (C)	3 medium	0.9
Lime juice, fresh (C)	1 cup	

Name of Fruit	Size of Portion	Grams Fiber
Loganberries, frz. (C)	¾ cup	
Loquats, raw (A)	12 medium	0.6
Lychees, raw (C)	9 medium	
Mandarin orange, wtrpk (A/C)	¾ cup sections	
Mango, raw (A/C)	½ medium	0.8
Medlar, bletted	1 medium	3.0
Mulberries, raw (C)	1 cup	1.3
Nectarine, raw (A)	1, 1½" diam	0.5
Orange, raw (A/C)	1 medium, 2½" diam	0.6
Orange juice, unsw. (C)	½ cup	
Papayas, raw (A/C)	½ papaya or 1 cup	1.2
Passionfruit, raw	3 medium fruits	6.0
Peach, raw (A)	1 medium or 1 cup chunks	2.3
Peaches, dried (A)	2 halves	2.3
Peaches, canned, wtrpk (A)	½ cup	
Pears, raw	½ large or 1 small	1.5
Pears, dried	1 half	1.5
Pears, canned, wtrpk	½ cup	
Persimmon, native, raw	2 medium	
Pineapple, raw, fresh	¾ cup	0.6
Pineapple, canned wtrpk	⅓ cup chunks	
Pineapple juice, unsw	½ cup	
Plum, raw, 2" diameter	2 plums	0.8
Pomegranate, raw	½	
Prunes, dried (A)	3 medium	0.5
Prune juice, unsweetened	⅓ cup	

Name of Fruit	Size of Portion	Grams Fiber
Quinces, raw	1 medium	1.6
Raisins	2 tablespoons	
Raspberries, raw (C)	1 cup	3.7
Strawberries, raw, whole (C)	1¼ cup	1.0
Tangelos, raw (C)	1½ medium	
Tangerines	2½"diam. (A/C) 2	0.6
Watermelon chunks, raw (A)	1¼ cup chunks	0.6

DAIRY PRODUCT GROUP

You're allowed TWO portions from this list daily.

This group consists of milk and products made from milk, with varying amounts of fat content. If yogurt or cheese is made from whole milk, the fat content stays the same. Only the lactose is destroyed by fermentation; the fat remains to contribute the same amount of unwanted extra calories as before.

Regular whole milk can have almost 4 percent fat, or as little as 3¼ percent in content. That type of milk product is too high in fat calories for the slimming portion of your program. Skim and very low-fat milk (½ percent or 1 percent) has very little fat and will be the only type of milk used during the slimming phase of the program. Once maintenance is reached, all forms of milk products will be allowed.

So-called "low-fat milk" has about 2 percent fat and is not allowed while you are trying to lose weight. Some of the milk products listed here are considered as fats or meat products, rather than as milk items. For example, cheeses are considered in the meat group because of their high protein content.

You'll notice that many milk items are not listed here. That's because they're forbidden during the slimming phase of the program. Those will be listed, with their exchange rates and other information, during the maintenance portion of the program.

The approximate cholesterol and sodium contents of each portion are listed in the following table. Mgc in the table refers to the milligrams of cholesterol per serving. Mgs refers to the milligrams of sodium per serving.

Food Name	Portion Size	Mgc	Mgs
Buttermilk from skim	1 cup	7.8	280
Butter—Not considered a milk portion; see fat portion list.			
Cheese—Usually considered with the meat-like foods; see meat protein list.			
Coffee whitener—Use fat free or nonfat whiteners.			
Cottage cheese—See meat-protein list.			
Cream—See fat portion list.			
Cream cheese—See fat portion list.			
Evaporated milk, skim	½ cup	4.0	148
Margarine—See fat portion list.			
Nonfat milk, dry	⅓ cup powder	5.0	145
Nonfat milk, mixed	1 cup	5.0	145
Milk, skim	1 cup	4.0	126
Milk, ½%	1 cup	7.0	123
Milk, 1%	1 cup	10.0	123
Tofu-based frozen desserts—Avoid, have added sugar.			
Yogurt, plain non-fat	½ cup	7.0	80
Yogurt, plain, with added non-fat milk solids	½ cup	2.0	87
Yogurt, flavored—Avoid usually. Has added sugars (see note below).			
Yogurt			
frozen—Avoid usually. Also has added sugars.			
Yogurt flavored with NutraSweet added —	1 cup		

(Kroger, Yoplait, Weight Watchers, Dannon, and Lite N'Lively: one cup equals about 100 calories).

For those last five yogurt items, even the flavored ones are allowed, because of the use of ½ percent milk products and NutraSweet. If you use any of the five brands, each serving counts as a low-fat milk AND a fruit portion.

SUBSTITUTION FOR DAIRY PRODUCTS

If you do not eat dairy products, you can compensate by adding two portions of meat and protein category foods to your daily allowance. In addition, you should take 1000 mg. of calcium (unless you have a medical condition where calcium supplements are not advised; check with your physician if you have a question about taking a calcium supplement).

VEGETABLE PORTION GROUP

You should have TWO items from this list every day.

At least one should be a good source of vitamins A and C. You probably noticed in the bread-pasta-cereal group that some food items traditionally thought of as vegetables are grouped with breads and pasta. That is because those vegetables — like corn, potatoes, yams, squash, and lima beans — are higher in starch content. While they might be vegetables biologically, nutritionally they're considered starches, just like bread or cereal.

A good rule, but one that has exceptions listed, is to think of foods derived from the stems, leaves, or pods of a plant as vegetable foods. Root and seed foods are most often starches that belong in the bread and cereal group.

Eat fresh and frozen vegetables whenever possible. Canned vegetables tend to have higher sodium content. Certain vegetables are high in sodium in any state, including raw; these are marked in the food lists.

Vegetables high in vitamin A and/or C are marked just like the items in the fruit list.

Vegetables that have almost no available calories when eaten raw are marked with an asterisk (*) as a free food. They may usually be eaten in reasonable quantities and not accounted for, if they are either raw or steamed for less than five minutes in a stovetop or counter-top steamer. Do NOT use a microwave steamer for steaming free vegetables; it cooks them too thoroughly.

If the vegetable is steamed for longer than five minutes, or cooked completely, it counts as a fully cooked vegetable portion and is no longer a free food. The cooking process, if done long enough, breaks down the cellulose and other complex carbohydrates into a digestible, and therefore accountable, food with usable calories for the body.

Some vegetables are rarely used for anything except salad material and are almost never cooked. When those are listed, the amount per serving is given as unlimited and it is assumed that they are not cooked.

When the asterisk-marked vegetables are uncooked or lightly steamed they are considered free foods. Those low-density free foods give people, on a calorie-restricted diet, an opportunity to feel "full" and not as "deprived" as they might otherwise feel. The bonus in extra dietary fiber can help insure bowel regularity, not to mention the other real benefits of extra fiber, vitamins, and minerals.

This program is used in the United Kingdom, so you'll see some vegetables listed that might not be available in the United States.

Food Name	Amount per serving if fully cooked
Alfalfa sprouts*	Unlimited
Artichoke, French or globe*	½ cup or ½ medium
Artichoke, Jerusalem*	½ cup
Asparagus* (A/C)	½ cup
Aubergine (eggplant)	½ cup
Avocado—See fat portion list; not counted as a vegetable.	
Bamboo shoots or sprouts*	¾ cup
Beans—See bread-cereal-pasta list; not counted as a vegetable.	
Bean sprouts*	½ cup
Beets (Beetroots)	½ cup
Beet greens*	½ cup (Not usually steamed)
Bokchoy (Chinese cabbage) (A/C)	½ cup
Broccoli* (A/C)	½ cup
Brussels sprouts* (C)	½ cup
Cabbage* all types (C)	½ cup
Carrots (A)	½ cup
Cauliflower* (C)	½ cup
Celeriac* (root celery)	1 cup (high in sodium)
Celery*	1 cup (high in sodium)
Chard*	Unlimited

Food Name	Amount per serving if fully cooked
Bean sprouts*	½ cup
Beets (Beetroots)	½ cup
Beet greens*	½ cup (not steamed)
Broccoli* (A/C)	½ cup
Brussels sprouts* (C)	½ cup
Cabbage* all types (C)	½ cup
Carrots (A)	½ cup
Cauliflower* (C)	½ cup
Celeriac* (root celery)	1 cup (high in sodium)
Celery*	1 cup (high in sodium)
Chard*	Unlimited
Bokchoy (Chinese cabbage) (A/C)	½ cup
Chicory* (A)	Unlimited
Chilies*	Unlimited
Chinese leaves* (A/C)	½ cup
Chives* (A/C)	Unlimited
Cilantro or Coriander*	Unlimited
Collard greens or tops*(C)	½ cup
Corn—See bread-cereal-pasta list; not counted as a vegetable	
Courgettes (Zucchini)* (A/C)	½ cup
Cress*	Unlimited
Cucumber*	Unlimited
Dandelion greens or tops*	Unlimited
Eggplant	½ cup
Endive*	Unlimited
Escarole* (A)	Unlimited

Food Name	Amount per serving if fully cooked
Fennel* (A)	Unlimited
Garlic	Use in reasonable amount
Green beans	½ Cup
Green onion tops*	Unlimited
Green peas (Petits Pois)	½ Cup
Green peppers* (C)	½ Cup
Kale* (A/C)	½ Cup
Kohlrabi, turnip cabbage (C)	½ Cup
Laverbread	½ Cup
Leeks(C)	½ Cup
Lettuce, all kinds	Unlimited
Mangetout*	½ Cup
Marrow* (A/C)	½ Cup
Mint*	Unlimited
Mushrooms*	½ Cup (not steamed)
Mustard greens or tops* (C)	½ Cup
Okra, "ladies fingers"*	½ Cup
Onions	½ Cup
Parsley* (A/C)	Unlimited
Peas, shelled—See bread-cereal-pasta list; not counted as vegetable	
Pea pods, Chinese Peas	½ Cup
Peas English or green	½ Cup
Pimentos*	½ Cup
Poke*	½ Cup
Pumpkin (A)	½ cup
Radishes*	

Food Name	Amount per serving if fully cooked
Red peppers* (C)	½ Cup
Rhubarb*	½ Cup
Romaine lettuce*	Unlimited
Rutabaga	½ Cup
Salsify*	Unlimited
Sauerkraut	½ cup (High in sodium)
Seakale*	Unlimited
Shallots	½ cup
Spinach* (A/C)	½ cup
Spring greens* (A/C)	½ cup
Spring onions*	Unlimited
Squash, summer* (A/C)	½ cup
Squash, crookneck* (A/C)	½ cup
String beans	½ cup
Tomato, fresh (A/C)	1 large
Tomato / Vegetable juice	½ cup (High in sodium)
Turnips	½ cup
Turnip greens (A/C)	½ cup
Water chestnuts	4 medium
Watercress* (A)	Unlimited
Waxbeans and other pod beans	½ cup
Zucchini squash* (A/C)	½ cup

MEAT AND PROTEIN GROUP

Women over 68 inches tall and all men are to have SEVEN portions from this food group daily.

Women 68 inches or shorter are allowed FIVE daily portions from this group.

For purposes of the list, all high protein foods will be referred to as meat, even though they may be fish, fowl, dairy, or other. It is difficult for someone on a diet to learn what constitutes a meat-like food and how to calculate values of a meat portion.

The foods listed here are marked according to whether there is a low, medium, or high content of fat in each portion. Each portion has about seven grams of protein, but the fat content varies from three grams per low-fat portion, to five grams per medium-fat portion, all the way up to eight grams of fat in each of the high-fat portions. That gives each portion 55, 75, or 100 calories, depending on the amount of fat contained in the protein food.

The weights given are for lean cuts, with all fat, bones and skin trimmed off prior to cooking. Four ounces of raw meat will usually weigh three ounces when cooked. To assist in making accurate decisions as to fat content, the low-fat protein foods are marked with two asterisks (**) and the moderate-fat ones with one asterisk (*); those with a high fat content are not marked at all.

Limit your choices in the high fat group to no more than three portions a week. If cholesterol is a problem, it's usually better to have no more than two eggs a week.

During the weight reduction phase of this program, severely limit the consumption of canned meats and fatty meat pies because of their extremely high fat content. Cheese and other fermented milk products are a good source of protein and calcium, but the fat content must be carefully considered in your selection of these foods.

Each quantity listed below is equal to one meat or meat-like portion. All weights given are cooked weights, with the cooking done in the appropriate way, using or retaining minimal fat in the cooking process. One ounce is also equal to 28 grams of boneless, trimmed weight. Some foods are higher in sodium and are marked with a capital "S" to signify that fact.

Remember, two asterisks (**) means low fat, and one asterisk (*) means moderate fat.

Food Name	Amount per Portion
Abalone**	1⅓ oz.
Anchovies, canned, drained** S	1 oz. or 9 fillets
Bacon-Not counted as a meat; see fat portion list.	
Bass**	1½ oz.
Beef, good or choice, lean*	1 oz.

Food Name	Amount per Portion
Beef flank, round, & sirloin*	1 oz.
Beef tenderloin*	1 oz.
Chipped beef* S	1 oz.
Beef, prime grades (ribs)	1 oz.
Beef, corned S	1 oz.
Beef, brisket, lean and fat*	1 oz.
Beef, forerib, lean*	1 oz.
Beef, ground, lean, drained*	1 oz.
Beef liver, kidney, tongue	1 oz.
Beef heart, brains	1 oz.
Beef, lean rump steak, grilled*	1 oz.
Beef, roasts and steaks*	1 oz.
Beef meatloaf	1 oz.
Canadian bacon	1 slice ¼ " thick by 3" diameter
Cheese, American S	1 oz.
Cheese, blue, Monterey, Swiss S	1 oz.
Cheese, cheddar S	1 oz.
Cheese, cottage, low-fat*	¼ cup
Cheese, cottage, 4% milk fat	¼ cup
Cheese, Edam, Gruyere*	1 oz.
Cheese, Parmesan, grated	2 tablespoons
Cheese, diet* S	1 oz. of less than 55 cal/oz. cheese
Cheese, farmer's, hoop, or pot**	¼ cup
Cheese, Mozzarella*	1 oz.
Cheese, ricotta*	¼ cup
Chicken, light or dark meat**	1 oz. without skin
Chicken with skin*	1 oz.

Food Name	Amount per Portion
Chicken livers, heart, or gizzard	1 oz.
Clams, raw** (S)	2 oz.
Cod**	1 oz.
Cold cuts, regular type (S)	1 slice, $\frac{1}{8}$" thick x 4½" diameter
Cold cuts, 86% fat-free (S)	1 oz. or 1 slice
Cold cuts, 95% fat-free (S)	1 oz. or 1 slice
Cornish hen, without skin**	1 oz.
Crabmeat, canned or fresh** (S)	2 oz. steamed
Duck, wild, without skin**	1 oz.
Duck, domestic, without skin*	1 oz.
Eggs, cooked any way without fat*	1 egg
Egg whites**	3 whites (from 3 eggs)
Egg substitutes, 55 cal./2 oz.	2 oz. or ¼ cup
Egg substitutes 56-80 cal./oz.	¼ cup
Fish, all types not specified*	1 oz. not fried or breaded
Fish, fried without grease	1 oz.
Flounder**	1 oz.
Frankfurter, beef and/or pork (S)	1 (10/lb.) give up 1 fat per portion
Frankfurter, chicken or turkey (S)	1 (10/lb.)
Goose, without skin, wild**	1 oz.
Goose, domestic, without skin*	1 oz.
Haddock or halibut**	1 oz.
Ham, fresh, lean*	1 oz.
Ham, canned, cured, or boiled** (S)	1 oz.
Herring, uncreamed or smoked** (S)	1 oz.
Knockwurst, smoked (S)	1 oz.

Food Name	Amount per Portion
Lamb, lean, chop or roast**	1 oz.
Lamb patties (ground lamb)	1 oz.
Lobster, fresh or canned**	1 oz.
Luncheon meat (bologna, salami) (S)	1 oz. or 1 slice
Oysters	6 medium
Peanut butter	1 tablespoon
Pheasant, wild	1 oz.
Pork, lean chops or cutlets*	1 oz.
Pork, loin roast & Boston butt*	1 oz.
Pork sausage (S)	1 patty, 1/4" thick x 3" diameter
Pork spareribs	1 oz.
Rabbit	1 oz.
Salmon** (S)	1 oz. fresh, or 1 1/2 oz. canned
Sardines, well drained of oil*	2 medium
Sausage, Polish or Italian (S)	1 oz.
Scallops** (S)	3 medium or 1 1/2 oz.
Shrimp, fresh or canned** (S)	2 oz. or 6 shrimp
Soy beans, cooked	1/4 cup
Squirrel**	1 oz.
Tofu* (not frozen dessert)	1 portion 2 1/2" x 2 3/4" x 1"
Turkey, light or dark meat**	1 oz.
Tuna, water packed** (S)	1/4 cup
Veal, lean, loin cut, chops**	1 oz.
Veal cutlet, ground or cubed*	1 oz. unbreaded
Venison	1 oz.
Pork spareribs	1 oz.
Rabbit	1 oz.

Food Name	Amount per Portion
Salmon** S	1 oz. fresh, or 1½ oz. canned
Sardines, well-drained of oil*	2 medium
Sausage, Polish or Italian S	1 oz.
Scallops**S	3 medium or 1½ oz.
Shrimp, fresh or canned** S	2 oz. or 6 shrimp
Soy beans, cooked	¼ cup
Squirrel**	1 oz.
Tofu* (Not frozen dessert)	1 portion 2½" x 2¾ " x 1"
Turkey, light or dark meat**	1 oz.
Tuna, water packed** S	¼ cup
Veal, lean, loin cut, chops**	1 oz.
Veal cutlet, ground or cubed*	1 oz. unbreaded
Venison	1 oz.

FAT LIST

You may have ONE and ONLY ONE portion from the list below during the slimming phase of The Doctors' Clinic-30 Program.

Each portion, or serving, of a fat contains five grams of fat and about 45 calories. Because this type of food is highly concentrated, you should take extreme care in measuring each quantity.

Many of the foods contain larger amounts of sodium and will be marked as such. When there is insignificant sodium there will be no figure given in that column; avoid obviously salty items, even if no figures are noted for them.

The fats are from saturated (more solid) fatty acids and also from the unsaturated oily fats.

The more liquid a fat is, the greater the proportion of unsaturated fats it contains.

Many fat items are not listed here, but will be listed in the chapter about the maintenance portion of the program.

Food Name	Size of Portion	Mg. Sodium
Avocado, 4" diameter	1/8 avocado (Fla. or Calif.)	
Butter	1 teaspoon	41
Butter, sweet, unsalted	1 teaspoon	
Cream, sour	2 tablespoons	
Cream, sour, substitute	1 oz. (Encore brand)	
Cream cheese	1 tablespoon	
Margarine, liquid	1 teaspoon	37
Margarine, stick	1 teaspoon	41
Margarine, stick, unsalt.	1 teaspoon	
Margarine, imit., diet	1 tablespoon	46
Mayonnaise, red. calorie	1 tablespoon	75
Oil (all types)	1 teaspoon	
Salad dressing, mayo, DIET	1 tablespoon	100
Salad dressing, all types	1 tablespoon	
Salad dressing, reduced calories — See free foods group.		

A low-fat diet is usually perceived as somewhat "dry" and unpalatable. Because fats are dense foods, with a lot of calories concentrated into a small volume, the addition of small amounts of fat into the daily intake does a lot to make the foods more pleasant to consume.

FREE FOODS

You don't have to keep track of free foods, except where there is an amount following the name of the product. Certain vegetable foods are marked as being permitted in unlimited amounts, only if the vegetable is raw, or lightly steamed. Also, remember to refer to the vegetable list for additional free foods, which are listed there.

Food Name
Bouillon or broth, without fat (better as low-sodium)
Candy, hard, sugar-free (two small pieces daily)

Food Name

Carbonated drinks, sugar-free Catsup, non-diet (one teaspoon daily)

Catsup, diet or imitation (two teaspoons daily)

Chili sauce, diet, Featherweight or similar brand (two teaspoons daily)

Cocoa powder, unsweetened (one tablespoon daily)

Coffee

Cranberries, unsweetened or with artificial sweeteners (½ cup daily)

Drink mixes, sugar-free (such as Crystal Lite, Kool Aid)

Extract of almond, lemon, chocolate, or vanilla (total of two tablespoons daily)

Gelatin, unflavored

Gelatin, sugar-free

Gum, sugar-free (2 pieces daily)

Hot sauce (two teaspoons daily)

Horseradish, plain, not the creamy mixtures Jam or jelly, sugar-free (two teaspoons daily)

Molly McButter Mustard

Pancake syrup, sugar-free (two tablespoons daily)

Pickles, dill, unsweetened Rhubarb, unsweetened (½ cup daily)

Salad dressing, low-calorie (maximum of 25 calories a day)

Taco sauce (two tablespoons)

Tea

Tonic water, sugar-free (careful: some brands are sweetened!)

Vinegar. Try the Balsamic variety of vinegar, diluted with water, and spiced up with a small amount of artificial sweetener and spices. It makes an excellent salad dressing.

These free foods are useful in filling out your daily intake and making things more interesting and tasty.

SPICES USED IN COOKING

The following spices are also permitted in reasonable amounts with the foods listed.

Spice	
Artichokes	bay leaves, marjoram, thyme.
Asparagus	caraway seed, mustard, nutmeg, sesame seed, tarragon.
Beans, green	basil, bay leaves, cloves, curry, dill, marjoram, mustard, nutmeg, oregano, j program savory, sesame seeds, tarragon, thyme.
Beans, lima	celery seed, chili powder, curry, oregano, sage.
Beets	allspice, bay leaves, caraway seeds, cloves, ginger.
Broccoli	caraway seed, marjoram, mustard, oregano, tarragon.
Brussels sprouts	caraway seed, mustard, nutmeg, sage.
Cabbage	allspice, basil, caraway seed, celery seed, cumin, curry powder, dill, fennel, mustard, nutmeg, oregano, savory, tarragon.
Carrots	allspice, bay leaves, caraway seed, celery seed, chives, cinnamon, cloves, curry, dill, ginger, mace, marjoram, mint, nutmeg, savory, tarragon, thyme.
Cauliflower	caraway seed, cayenne, celery seed, curry, dill, marjoram, mustard, nutmeg, oregano, paprika, rosemary, savory, tarragon.
Com	cayenne, celery seed, chili powder, chives, curry, paprika.
Eggplant	allspice, basil, bay leaves, chili powder, marjoram, sage, thyme.
Mushrooms	marjoram, rosemary, tarragon, thyme.
Onions	basil, bay leaves, caraway seed, chili powder, curry, ginger, mustard, nutmeg, oregano, paprika, sage, thyme.
Peas	basil, chili powder, dill, marjoram, mint, mustard, oregano, poppy seed, rosemary, sage.

Spice	
Potatoes, Sweet	allspice, cardamom, cinnamon, cloves, ginger, nutmeg, poppy seed.
Potatoes, white	basil, bay leaves, caraway seed, celery seed, chives, dill, fennel, mace, mustard, oregano, paprika, rosemary, savory, sesame seed, thyme.
Spinach	allspice, basil, cinnamon, dill, mace, marjoram, nutmeg, oregano, rosemary, sesame seed.
Summer Squash	basil, bay leaves, cardamom, mace, marjoram, mustard, rosemary.
Winter Squash	allspice, basil, cardamom, cinnamon, cloves, ginger, marjoram, nutmeg, paprika.
Tomatoes	basil, bay leaves, caraway seed, celery seed, chili powder, cloves, curry, dill, garlic, marjoram, oregano, rosemary, sage, savory, sesame seed, thyme.
Turnips	allspice, caraway seed, celery seed, dill, oregano.

WHAT ABOUT A VEGETARIAN REDUCING DIET?

It is possible to lose weight on a vegetarian diet, but the caloric costs to consume the required daily amount of protein are higher when meat, fish, and poultry items are excluded. It is even harder when egg and/or milk products are not consumed. Please refer to the original Clinic-30 Program lists.

FOR TRUE VEGANS, THE FOLLOWING FOOD ITEMS ARE ALLOWED EACH DAY:

- Bread-Starch Group, 7 serving a day. This includes those starches and starchy vegetables that are in the initial diet and are not made with milk products. Use the serving sizes that are listed for each food in your count.
- Fruit Group, 4 serving a day. Identical list with The Clinic-30 Program. The fully cooked vegetables are from the same source.
- Fully cooked Vegetables, 4 serving a day. Free vegetables are the same as on The Clnic-30 Program and are in unlimited amounts if raw or lightly steamed.

78

- Meat alternative Group, 4 servings for women and 6 servings for men, and women over 70 inches in height. A serving would be ½ cup cooked beans or peas, 2 tablespoons low-fat peanut butter, 3 ounces tofu, ¼ cup nuts or seeds, or 2 ounces textured vegetable protein product.
- Vegetable fats and oils. Omit while on the reducing phase of this diet.
- Free foods remain the same as on The Clinic-30 Program.

LACTO-OVA VEGETARIANS, THE FOLLOWING ITEMS ARE ALLOWED EACH DAY:

- Bread starch Group is the same, except now you can include those in the group that are cooked or baked with milk and/or eggs.
- Fruit Group is the same.
- Fully Cooked Vegetable Group is the same. Free Foods, including raw and highly lightly steamed vegetables are the same.
- Meat Alternative Group is the same with the addition of the white of one egg being one serving and 1½ ounce fat-free cheese product, or ¼ cup low-fat or fat-free cottage cheese also being a serving in this group. Use any of the milk selections on the low-fat milk list of The Clinic-30 Program as a serving of a meat alternative.

When a vegetarian reaches his or her weight goal, the same framework of foods is used, but more food is gradually added until a balance between calories in and calories out exists.

CHAPTER SEVEN

MAINTAINING YOUR SLIMMER FIGURE

"You can't expect to see change if you never do anything differently" – Meg Biram

Now what? Once you reach your weight goal, what do you do next?

First, understand that this is one of the most dangerous times in your weight reduction program. Once you reach your desired weight, it's very easy to think, "I'm cured. I never have to worry about my weight again. I did it!"

A colleague, Dr. Richard Stuart, has labeled this point in the weight loss program as the "Ah Hah!" point; it's the time when you might erroneously cry out: "Ah Hah! I've arrived at my desired weight. Now I can eat again!"

All the good habits you've acquired, all the information on good nutrition you've learned, all the work you've done up to this point cannot end. You must continue to have good eating, shopping, and cooking practices for the rest of your life. If you're not willing to accept that fact, then you need to re-evaluate your motivation for wanting to lose weight.

When you lose weight, it's not like getting over an upper respiratory infection. The obesity problem is still there; it's just buried under some newly learned habits. If permanent weight control is the object of your efforts, you must change many bad habits and restructure the entire mental state that caused the problem of obesity in the first place.

The average person with a weight problem thinks like an overweight person. Taking even a significant amount of fat off that person's body, with diet alone, will do nothing to alter the thinking patterns. It takes a lot of work to maintain the desired weight, including changing attitudes and patterns of behavior.

You must continue to deal with saboteurs and feeders, and you must keep up your exercise and a pattern of increased activity.

You must change your thinking; model your behavior on that of people who are thin.

Thin people eat only when they are hungry.

Thin people never gorge themselves on anything.

Thin people pay attention to what their bodies are telling them, and they don't rely on external cues to tell them to eat.

When thin people have had enough to eat, they do not continue to eat, regardless if their plate or bowl still has food on it.

You must think like a thin person at all times. Never give in to fat thinking again. Mimic your thin friends and acquaintances in their behavior.

Don't deny your body the food it needs. Don't skip meals and produce a state of deprivation and hunger. The best appetite suppressant is good food in the proper amounts, usually in a pattern of three meals and three snacks a day.

Listen to what your body says to you. Avoid false hunger signals. Make sure that what you're feeling is really hunger and not just a desire for food or treats. Stress is NOT a signal to eat; neither is fatigue, boredom, anger, anxiety, depression, sleepiness, or happiness. When the body NEEDS food and the feeling is REALLY hunger, then you should eat.

Yes, you've worked hard to get to this point, but losing weight is only part of the battle. You have to maintain that weight loss for the rest of your life. And you'll do that through changing your behavior and habits; exercising; and eating right.

The foods you eat, and in what quantities, are still very important.

- You have to accept the following facts:

- You cannot eat all you want, and never will be able to eat all you want.

- You cannot eat all the kinds of food you want. Yes, you can eat some foods, even problem foods, occasionally, but never a steady diet of cookies or potato chips. Accept the fact that those days are over.

- You can eat in a fast-food restaurant now that you're starting maintenance; but you cannot eat there steadily, only occasionally.

- Your scales, measuring cups, measuring spoons, and ruler are still necessary tools as you go through the stabilization phase of this program. Until you've been on maintenance for at least two months, do not fry any of your foods, except if instructed in this program.

- It's still necessary to keep track of portion sizes in the six basic food groups. And you'll still be using the exchange system to maintain your weight.

USING THE EXCHANGE SYSTEM TO MAINTAIN YOUR WEIGHT

At the start of the last chapter, we figured out what your ideal weight should be, depending on your body size. We're going to use another formula here to determine what your "caloric intake" should be once you reach your ideal weight.

In other words, your caloric intake will change during the maintenance phase of this program; that means you'll be able to add food exchanges from the six groups — a fat exchange or two, a meat exchange or two, etc.

That gives you more food options, and will help you reach a good balance between the calories that you take in and those you burn.

Obviously, during the slimming phase, the goal is to burn off more calories each day than you took in.

In maintenance, the goal is to balance the two. You should not be losing or gaining any more weight.

Up to this point, you've used your clothing sizes to determine and monitor your fat loss; occasionally, you had to use your scale. Now, you must use your scale a little more frequently.

If you reach your ideal weight, but then start gaining, you know that you're out of balance. That means you're taking in more calories than you're burning, and you have to adjust. You may be eating too much, or not exercising enough, or both.

Likewise, if you're losing weight, you're also out of balance, and you must do something to restore that balance. Do not exercise as much, add more food, or both.

HOW MUCH SHOULD I EAT TO MAINTAIN MY WEIGHT?

The first thing you have to do is calculate your caloric needs, what I call "caloric intake"; this is never a perfect calculation, but it's close enough for our needs.

Women, multiply your goal body weight in pounds by 16. Thus, a 100-pound woman would multiply 100 X 16 to come up with 1600. That's the total caloric intake for a medium-frame woman, who weighs 100 pounds and wants to maintain her weight. However, the first week of maintenance, start at 25 percent less than the total caloric need. To continue with the original example, 1600 calories minus 25 percent (400 calories) equals 1200 calories.

Thus, a woman, who reaches her weight goal of 100 pounds, would start her first week of maintenance on a 1200-calorie diet. (Don't worry, you don't have to actually count calories. The exchange charts are broken down by total calories to make it easier.)

A man should multiply his ideal weight by 18. Thus, if his ideal weight is 170 pounds, he'd multiply 170 X 18 for 3,060. Then subtract 25 percent for the starting figure, and the man would have a maintenance diet of about 2300 calories during his first week.

Start at the figure that is 25 percent less than your caloric needs, and if you're still losing a little bit of weight, add 100 calories each week.

At the end of each week that you're still decreasing slightly in weight, add exchanges permitted from the next highest caloric chart. For example, on the 1400-calorie diet, you're permitted four portions from the bread-pasta-cereal group. On the 1500-calorie diet, you're permitted five portions from the bread group. So you would add one extra bread portion. The next week, if you're still losing a little weight, go to the next caloric level, adding one exchange at a time.

Eventually, you'll reach a level where your weight stays the same. Now you are in balance, and on true maintenance. When you reach that level, you'll know for sure how much food you need to eat to keep your new, slimmer figure.

If you exercise a little more, you can eat a little more. If you exercise a little less, then you'll have to eat a little less, or you'll gain weight.

PORTION LISTS FOR MAINTENANCE OF YOUR WEIGHT LOSS

1,200 calories	
Milk	two portions a day
Vegetables	two portions a day
Meat group	five portions a day
Fruit	three portions a day
Bread-starch	four portions a day
Fat group	two portions a day
Free foods	as desired, in moderation

1,400 calories	
Milk	two portions a day
Vegetables	three portions a day

1,400 calories

Meat group	six portions a day
Fruits	three portions a day
Bread-starch	four portions a day
Fat group	two portions a day
Free foods	as desired, in moderation

1,500 calories

Milk	two portions a day
Vegetables	three portions a day
Meat group	six portions a day
Fruits	three portions a day
Bread-starch	five portions a day
Fat group	two portions a day
Free foods	as desired, in moderation

1,600 calories

Milk	two portions a day
Vegetables	three portions a day
Meat group	six portions a day
Fruits	three portions a day
Bread-starch	six portions a day
Fat group	three portions a day
Free foods	as desired, in moderation

1,800 calories

Milk	two portions a day
Vegetables	four portions a day
Meat group	seven portions a day

1,800 calories

Fruits	three portions a day
Bread-starch	seven portions a day
Fat group	three portions a day
Free foods	as desired, in moderation

2,000 calories

Milk	two portions a day
Vegetables	four portions a day
Meat group	eight portions a day
Fruits	four portions a day
Bread-starch	eight portions a day
Fat group	three portions a day
Free foods	as desired, in moderation

2,200 calories

Milk	two portions a day
Vegetables	four portions a day
Meat group	nine portions a day
Fruits	four portions a day
Bread-starch	nine portions a day
Fat group	four portions a day
Free foods	as desired, in moderation

2,400 calories

Milk	three portions a day
Vegetables	four portions a day
Meat group	nine portions a day
Fruits	four portions a day

2,400 calories

Bread-starch	nine and one-half portions
Fat group	four portions a day
Free foods	as desired, in moderation

2,600 calories

Milk	three portions a day
Vegetables	four portions a day
Meat group	10 portions a day
Fruits	four portions a day
Bread-starch	11 portions a day
Fat group	four portions a day
Free foods	as desired, in moderation

2,800 calories

Milk	three portions a day
Vegetables	four portions a day
Meat group	11 portions a day
Fruits	five portions a day
Bread-starch	12 portions a day
Fat group	four portions a day
Free foods	as desired, in moderation

3,000 calories

Milk	three portions a day
Vegetables	four portions a day
Meat group	12 portions a day
Fruits	five portions a day
Bread-starch	13 portions a day

3,000 calories	
Fat group	four portions a day
Free foods	as desired, in moderation

Use these portion lists just like the ones you used during the slimming phase. Once you calculate your caloric needs, you can start at the level that is 25 percent below your needs. Then work yourself up to the point where your weight stays balanced with what you eat.

Refer to the food lists in the previous chapters to find the exchange values and portion sizes.

Build your own menus for breakfast, lunch, and dinner. Do you have a lot of physical work to do in the day? Then use more exchanges in breakfast and lunch, and fewer in dinner.

The maintenance part of this program is as flexible as the slimming part, and just as easy to follow.

A meal plan for a man on a 2,200-calorie maintenance program might look like this:

Breakfast	Lunch
one milk portion	three meat portions
one meat portion	two vegetable portions
two bread portions	three bread portions
two fruit portions	one fat portion
one fat portion	one fruit portion

Dinner	Snacks
one milk portion	one milk portion
three meat portions	one bread portion
two bread portions	two fruit portions
two vegetable portions	
one fat portion	

Also, some foods that were forbidden during the slimming phase can now be eaten, but only occasionally and in moderation.

Those foods are listed here, with their portion sizes. Again, these can only be eaten once you reach your goal weight, not before. (Use these lists in conjunction with the previous lists.)

FRUIT AND FRUIT-LIKE ITEMS

Food Name	Size of Portion
Molasses, blackstrap	
Honey	1 tablespoon
Fructose	1 tablespoon

For all three of the above, use only a single portion of any one of them a day, more than that is just too much for you to have, at least for the first year on maintenance.

DAIRY PRODUCTS

Food Name	Portion Size	Mgc	Mgs
Buttermilk from 2%	1 cup	9.0	257
Evaporated milk, whole	½ cup	37.0	133
Goat's milk, 4.5% fat	1 cup	28.0	122
Milk, 2%	1 cup	18.0	122
Milk, whole	1 cup	35.0	119
Soybean milk	1 cup		55
Soybean milk-Soyamel	1 cup		190
Ice cream, no sugar added*	1 cup		
Yogurt, frozen, TCBY	5 oz. cup (With Aspartame or Nutrasweet and no sugar added.)		
Yogurt, frozen, Freshens	5 oz. cup (With Aspartame or Nutrasweet and no sugar added.)		

*Use the Edy's brand; any of the following flavors: Butter pecan, Chips 'N Swirls, All About PB, Double Fudge Brownie, Mint Chocolate Chips, Neapolitan, Strawberry, Vanilla, Triple Chocolate, Chocolate Fudge, Raspberry Vanilla Swirl, Vanilla Chocolate Swirl, or Vanilla 'N Caramel. There may be other brands of no sugar added ice cream, but Edy's was the only one that sent *me nutritional information.*

FATS & OILS GROUP

Food Name	Size of Portion	Mgs
Almonds, dry roasted	6 whole unsalted nuts	
Bacon, fried, drained	1 slice	200
Beamaise sauce	1 teaspoon	60
Brazil nuts, dry roasted	2 medium, unsalted nuts	
Caraway seeds	2 tablespoons	
Cashews, dry roasted	1 tablespoon, unsalted nuts	
Chitterlings, cooked	½ ounce	
Chocolate, unsw., melted	2 teaspoons	
Chocolate, bitter	⅓ oz. or ⅓ square	
Coconut, shredded	2 tablespoons	29
Coffee whitener, liquid	2 tablespoons	
Coffee whitener, powder	4 teaspoons	
Cream (light, coffee, table)	2 tablespoons	
Cream, whipping, heavy	1 tablespoon	
Filberts, dry roasted	5 nuts, unsalted	
Hazelnuts, dry roasted	5 nuts, unsalted	
Hollandaise sauce	1 teaspoon	28
Mayonnaise	1 teaspoon	26
Nuts, mixed or others	1 tablespoon dry roasted, unsalted nuts	
Olives	10 small, 5 large (Lots of sodium)	
Peanuts, dry roasted	20 small or 10 large, unsalted	
Pecans, dry roasted	2 whole, 4 halves, unsalted	
Pumpkin seeds, dry roasted	2 teaspoons, unsalted	

Food Name	Size of Portion	Mgs
Salt pork	¼ oz. cube	
Seeds, dry roasted (no shells)	1 tablespoon, unsalted	
Tartar sauce	1 teaspoon	60
Walnuts, dry roasted	2 whole, unsalted	

One of the biggest complaints I hear about other programs is that many soups, prepared, and frozen foods are hard to figure into the diet and maintenance plan. We do live in a fast-paced society, and I know people are going to grab a can of soup and heat it for lunch or dinner. The problem is, you cannot figure the food values of the item into your daily allotment.

For example, do you count a can of vegetable beef soup as one meat exchange, one vegetable exchange, or a bread exchange. (The answer: it's one-half of a bread exchange, and one meat exchange.)

The following lists allow you to enjoy some of the pre-packaged foods available today, while still adhering to your maintenance plan.

Those items are not allowed during your slimming phase, but you may eat them now, and you should figure their food values into your daily allotment.

Here are exchange values for many, many prepared foods. I've also included the exchange values for certain alcoholic beverages. Now that you're on maintenance, you can have a drink now and then. However, you need to account for the food value in your daily allotment.

ALCOHOL

BEER

Type	Serving size	Exchange information
Ale, Mild	8 oz.	1½ fat, 1 fruit
Beer	8 oz.	1½ fat, 1 fruit

WINES

Type	Serving size	Exchange Information
Champagne, Brut	3 oz.	1⅔ fat
Champagne, Extra dry	3 oz.	1⅔ fat, ½ fruit

Type	Serving size	Exchange Information
Dubonnet	3 oz.	1½ fat, 1 fruit
Dry Marsala	3 oz.	2 fat, 2 fruit
Sweet Marsala	3 oz.	2 fat, 2½ fruit
Muscatel	4 oz.	2⅓ fat, 1½ fruit
Port	4 oz.	2⅓ fat, 1½ fruit
Dry Red Wine	3 oz.	1⅔ fat
Sake	3 oz.	1 fat, 1 fruit
Domestic Sherry	3½ oz.	1½ fat, ½ fruit
Dry vermouth	3½ oz.	2⅔ fat, 1 fruit
Sweet vermouth	3½ oz.	2⅔ fat, 1 fruit
Dry white wine	3 oz.	1½ fat

LIQUEURS AND CORDIALS

Type	Serving Size	Exchange Information
Amaretto	1 oz.	1⅓ fat, 1½ fruit
Crème de Cacao	1 oz.	1½ fat, 1 fruit
Crème de Menthe	1 oz.	1½ fat, 1 fruit
Curacao	1 oz.	1½ fat, 1 fruit
Drambuie	1 oz.	1½ fat, 1 fruit
Tia Maria	1 oz.	1½ fat, 1 fruit

SPIRITS

Bourbon, brandy, cognac, Canadian whiskey, gin, rye, rum, Scotch, tequila, and vodka are essentially free of carbohydrates. Caloric or fat portion count depends on the proof. Values are rounded off.

Type	Serving size	Exchange Information
80 proof	1 oz.	1½ fat

Type	Serving size	Exchange Information
84 proof	1 oz.	1½ fat
90 proof	1 oz.	1⅔ fat
94 proof	1 oz.	2 fat
97 proof	1 oz.	2 fat
100 proof	1 oz.	2¼ fat

HOW TO DEAL WITH A CANNED OR PACKAGED FOOD THAT IS NOT LISTED BELOW:

The food industry is constantly changing its products. The lists prepared from today's data may be totally inadequate a week from now to determine the exchange count.

Let's examine the Nutrition Facts label of a can of Split Pea and Ham soup put out by Healthy Choice.

The first thing we look at is the serving size, usually given in terms of fluid ounces, measuring cups, etc. Then look at the serving per container. Sometimes the serving may be 50 calories, but the container has six servings, meaning the entire can or bottle or box has 300 calories, not 50.

After you have gotten the serving size, look at the number of calories per serving and the calories from fat. Don't be shocked to see that fat in some food items is more than half the calories. The Healthy Choice soup in question has 2 servings per can, each one being 8 ounces. There are 150 calories per serving, of which 15 calories (or 10%) is from fat; that is not a bad percentage. If you come across something with more than 30% fat calories, use it with great caution, unless you wish to calculate it as part of your allowed fat intake. The 30% or less fat calorie content is preferred.

The total fat is the next item on a nutrition label. This soup has 2 grams of fat, of which only 0.5 grams is saturated fat; this is a good food. The saturated fat is listed separately from the total fat content, a good step in preventing deceptive advertising, which unfortunately occurs at times.

There are fewer than 5milligrams of cholesterol in each serving of this soup, and the sodium content per serving is 480 milligrams. The sodium is somewhat high, 20% of a person's daily needs (if a person is on a 2, 000 calorie diet).

There are 25 grams total carbohydrates per serving, of which 2 grams are sugars and 3 grams are fiber; the rest is starch and related complex carbohydrates. Twenty grams of complex carbohydrates would be about 80 calories, or slightly over the amount in a serving of bread. There are 12 grams of protein, or about½ serving of meat. The actual count on the label - and I appreciate Healthy Choice doing this counting - is½ bread portions and½ meat portion.

You can do the same thing. Take the number of calories of bread-like foods and starches (grams x 4 = calories) and divide by 80 to get the number of bread-starch portions per serving. Take the calories of protein (also grams x 4) and divide by 80 to get the number of meat or meat-like portions.

There are a lot of frozen "diet" entrees out there with more coming into stores each month. Some of the frozen entrees may not have the exact portion lists on the package, so I developed an alternative way for you to count the portions. Avoid those "hearty portion" entrees with more than 300 calories per serving.

- For 220 calories, deduct 2 breads and 1 meat portion.
- For 240 calories, deduct 2 breads, 1 meat and 1 cooked vegetable.
- For 260 calories, deduct 2 breads, 1 meat and 2 cooked vegetables.
- For 300 calories, deduct 2 breads, 2 meats and 1 cooked vegetable.
- For 350 calories, deduct 3 breads, 2 meats and 2 cooked vegetables.

You deduct bread, meat, or vegetable portions from your daily ration, even if there is no bread, meat, or vegetable in the entrée. Trust me, it comes out accurately for your daily caloric needs.

If you still have trouble figuring out the food portions for a certain item, write that company or call them (most have addresses and phone numbers on the container) for further help.

CANNED AND PACKAGED FOODS

AUNT PENNY'S SAUCES

Food Name	Serving Size	Exchange Information
Aunt Penny's Cheese Sauce	2 tablespoons	½ meat, ½ vegetable
Aunt Penny's Hollandaise Sauce	2 tablespoons	½ meat, ½ vegetable
Aunt Penny's White Sauce	2 tablespoons	½ meat, ½ vegetable

BANQUET BRAND

Food Name	Serving Size	Exchange Information

Food Name	Serving Size	Exchange Information
Beef Stew	8 oz.	2 bread, 1 meat
Chicken and Dumplings	8 oz.	2 bread, 3 meat
Creamed Chipped Beef	5 oz.	1 meat, 2 vegetable
Salisbury Steak with Gravy	5 oz.	2 meat, 1 vegetable, 1 fat
Spaghetti with Meat Sauce	8 oz.	2 meat, 3 fruit, 1 fat

BETTY CROCKER

Food Name	Serving Size	Exchange Information
Macaroni and Cheddar	½ cup	1 bread and 1 fat
Noodles Almondine	½ cup	1 bread, 1 milk, ½ fat
Noodles Italiano	½ cup	1 bread, ½ milk
Noodles Romanoff	½ cup	1 bread, 1 milk, ½ fat
Chili-Tomato Hamburger Helper Mix	⅕ package	2 bread, ½ fat
Hamburger Helper Mix	⅕ package	1½ bread, trace fat
Lasagna Hamburger Helper Mix	⅕ package	2 bread
Spaghetti Hamburger Helper Mix	⅕ package	2 bread
Cheeseburger Macaroni Hamburger Helper Mix	⅕ package	2 bread, 1 fat
Rice Milanese	½ cup	2 bread, 1½ fat
Rice Provence	½ cup	2 breads, ½ fat
Creamy Noodles 'n Tuna or Hamburger Helper Mix	⅕ package	2 bread, 2 fat
Creamy Rice 'n Tuna or Hamburger Helper Mix	⅕ package	2 bread, 1 fat
Dry Hash Brown Potato Mix	¼ package	3 bread

Food Name	Serving Size	Exchange Information
Dry Scalloped Potato Mix	¼ package	3 bread
Instant Mashed Potato Buds	½ cup	1½ bread

BIRDS EYE BRAND

Food Name	Serving Size	Exchange Information
Awake Imitation Orange Juice	½ cup	1½ fruit
Bavarian-style Beans w/Spaetzle	½ cup	2 vegetable
Broccoli Spears in Butter Sauce	½ cup	½ vegetable and 1 fat
Broccoli w/Cheese Sauce	½ cup	2 vegetable and 2 fat
Broccoli, Carrots and Pasta Twists	½ cup	½ bread, 1 vegetable, 1 fat
Carrots w/Brown Sugar Glaze	½ cup	1 fruit, 1 vegetable, ½ fat
Chinese-Style Vegetables	½ cup	1 vegetable
Cool Whip Nondairy Topping	2 tablespoons	¼ milk
Corn in Butter Sauce	½ cup	1 bread and 1 fat
Corn, Green Beans & Pasta Curls	½ cup	1 bread, 1 vegetable, 1 fat
Corn, Peas, and Tomatoes	½ cup	2 vegetable
French-style Green Beans w/Almonds	½ cup	1 vegetable, ½ fat
French-style Green Beans w/Mushrooms	½ cup	1 vegetable
French-Style Rice	½ cup	1½ bread, 1 vegetable

Food Name	Serving Size	Exchange Information
Green Beans in Cream Sauce	½ cup	½ bread, 1 vegetable, 1½ fat
Green Peas and Onions	½ cup	2 vegetable
Green Peas in Butter Sauce	½ cup	1½ vegetable, 1 fat
Green Peas and Celery	½ cup	1½ vegetable
Green Peas and Mushrooms	½ cup	1½ vegetable
Italian-Style Vegetables	½ cup	2 vegetable
Italian-Style Rice	½ cup	1 vegetable, 1½ breads
Japanese-Style Vegetables	½ cup	2 vegetables
Mixed Vegetables w/Onion Sauce	½ cup	1 vegetable, ½ bread, 1 fat
New England-Style Vegetables	½ cup	1 vegetable, ½ bread, 1 fat
Oriental-Style Rice	½ cup	1 vegetable, 1½ bread
Peas, Shells, and Corn	½ cup	1 vegetable, 1 bread, 1 fat
Peas, Shells, and Mushrooms	½ cup	1 vegetable, 1 bread, 1 fat
Pennsylvania Dutch-style Vegetables	½ cup	1½ vegetable
Rice and Peas with Mushrooms	½ cup	1 vegetable, 1 bread
San Francisco-Style Vegetables	½ cup	2 vegetable
Spanish-Style Rice	½ cup	1 vegetable, 1½ bread
Creamed Spinach	½ cup	1 vegetable, 1 fat
Wisconsin Country-Style Vegetables	½ cup	1½ vegetable
Crinkle or Plain French Fried Potatoes	3 oz. (1 serving)	1½ breads, 1 fat

Food Name	Serving Size	Exchange Information
Potato Pattie	3 oz. (1 serving)	1 bread, 2 fat
Potato Puffs	⅓ package	1 bread, 2 fat
Hash Browns	½ cup	1 bread
Onion Rings	2 oz. (½ sm. pkg.) or 2 oz. (⅓ lg. pkg.)	1 bread, 2 fat

BOUNTY (CAMPBELL'S

Food Name	Serving Size	Exchange Information
Beef Stew	1 cup	1 bread, 2 meat
Chicken Stew	1 cup	1 bread, 1½ meat
Chili Con Carne w/Beans	1 cup	1 bread, 1 meat

CAMPBELL'S CONDENSED SOUPS

(All servings ½ can, given in number of prepared ounces)

Food Name	Serving Size	Exchange Information
Asparagus, Cream of	10 oz.	1 bread, 1 fat
Bean with Bacon	11 oz.	2 bread, ½ meat, 1 fat
Beef	11 oz.	1 bread, 1 meat
Beef Broth (bouillon)	10 oz.	Free Food
Beef Broth and Barley	11 oz.	1 bread, ½ fat
Beef Broth and Noodles	10 oz.	1 bread, ½ fat
Beef Noodle	10 oz.	1 bread, ½ fat
Beef Teriyaki	10 oz.	1 bread, ½ meat
Beefy Mushroom	10 oz.	½ bread, 1 meat
Black Bean	11 oz.	1½ bread, ½ meat
Celery, Cream of	10 oz.	½ bread, 2 fat

Food Name	Serving Size	Exchange Information
Cheddar Cheese	11 oz.	1 milk, 2 fat
Chicken Alphabet	10 oz.	1 bread, ½ fat
Chicken Broth	10 oz.	1 meat
Chicken Broth and Noodles	10 oz.	½ bread, 1 fat
Chicken Broth and Rice	10 oz.	1 bread
Chicken Broth and Vegetables	10 oz.	½ bread
Chicken, Cream of	10 oz.	½ bread, 2 fat
Chicken 'n Dumplings	10 oz.	½ bread, ½ meat, 1 fat
Chicken Gumbo	10 oz.	1 bread
Chicken Noodle	10 oz.	1 bread, ½ fat
Chicken Noodle O's	10 oz.	1 bread, ½ fat
Chicken with Rice	10 oz.	½ bread, 1 fat
Chicken with Stars	10 oz.	½ bread, 1 fat
Chicken Vegetable	10 oz.	1 bread, ½ fat
Chili Beef	11 oz.	1½ bread, 1 meat, ½ fat
Clam Chowder (Manhattan)	10 oz.	1 bread, ½ fat
Clam Chowder (New England made with milk)*	10 oz.	1 bread, 1 meat, 1 fat, ½ milk
Consomme (Beef)	10 oz.	1 vegetable
Creamy Chicken Mushroom	10 oz.	1 bread, 2 fat
Curly Noodle with Chicken	10 oz.	1 bread, ½ fat
Green Pea	11 oz.	2 bread, 1 meat, ½ fat
Meatball Alphabet	10 oz.	1 bread, 1 meat, ½ fat
Minestrone	10 oz.	1 bread, ½ fat
Mushroom, Cream of	10 oz.	1 bread, 1 fat
Mushroom, Golden	10 oz.	1 bread, 1 fat
Noodles & Ground Beef	10 oz.	1 bread, 1 fat

Food Name	Serving Size	Exchange Information
Onion	10 oz.	1 bread, ½ fat
Onion, Cream of (made with water and milk) *	10 oz.	1 bread, ½ fat, ½ milk
Oriental Chicken	10 oz.	1 vegetable, 1 fat
Oyster Stew (made with milk)*	10 oz.	½ bread, ½ meat, 1½ fat, ½ milk
Pepper Pot	10 oz.	1 bread, ½ meat, ½ fat
Potato, Cream of (made with water and milk)*	10 oz.	1 bread, 1 fat, ½ milk
Shrimp, Cream of (made with water and milk) *	10 oz.	1 bread, 2 fat, ½ milk
Split Pea with Ham and Bacon	11 oz.	2 bread, 1 meat, ½ fat
Tomato	10 oz.	1 vegetable, 1 bread, ½ fat
Tomato (made with milk) *	10 oz.	1 veg, 1 bread, 1½ fat, ½ milk
Tomato Bisque	11 oz.	2 bread, ½ fat
Tomato Rice, Old Fashioned	11 oz.	2 bread, ½ fat
Turkey Noodle	10 oz.	1 bread, ½ fat
Turkey Vegetable	10 oz.	1 bread, ½ fat
Vegetable	10 oz.	1 vegetable, 1 bread
Vegetable Beef	10 oz.	½ bread, 1 meat
Vegetable, Old Fashioned	10 oz.	1 bread, ½ fat
Vegetarian Vegetable	10 oz.	1 bread, ½ fat
Won Ton	10 oz.	½ bread, ½ meat

* Exchanges based on addition of whole milk

CAMPBELL'S SOUP FOR ONE

(All servings 1 can, given in prepared ounces)

Food Name	Serving Size	Exchange Information
Bean, Old Fashioned w/Ham	11 oz.	2 bread, ½ meat, 1 fat
Burly Vegetable Beef	11 oz.	1 vegetable, 1 bread, 1 meat
Clam Chowder (New England made with whole milk) *	11 oz.	1 bread, ½ meat, 1½ fat, ½ milk
Full Flavored Chicken Vegetable	11 oz.	1 bread, 1 fat
Golden Chicken & Noodles	11 oz.	1 bread, 1 fat
Mushroom, Cream of, savory	11 oz.	1 bread, 2 fat
Tomato Royale	11 oz.	2 bread, 1 fat
Vegetable, Old World	11 oz.	1 bread, 1 fat

* Exchanges based on addition of whole milk.

CAMPBELL'S CHUNKY SOUPS

(Individual service size, 1 can, undiluted oz.)

Food Name	Serving Size	Exchange Information
Chunky Beef	10¾ oz.	1½ bread, 1½ meat
Chunky Beef with Noodles (Stroganoff Style)	10¾ oz.	2 bread, 1½ meat, 2 fat
Chunky Chicken	10¾ oz.	1½ bread, 2 meat, ½ fat
Chunky Chili Beef	11 oz.	2½ bread, 2½ meat
Chunky Clam Chowder(Manhattan Style)	10¾ oz.	1½ bread, ½ meat, 1 fat
Chunky Ham'n Butter Bean	10¾ oz.	2 bread, 1½ meat, 1½ fat

Food Name	Serving Size	Exchange Information
Chunky Old Fashioned Bean w/Ham	11 oz.	2 bread, 1½ meat, 1 veg, 1½ fat
Chunky Old Fashioned Vegetable Beef	10 ¾ oz.	1 bread, 1 meat, 1 veg, ½ fat
Chunky Sirloin Burger	10½ oz.	1 bread, 1½ meat, 1 veg, 1 fat
Chunky Split Pea w/Ham	10¾ oz.	2 bread, 1 meat, 1 fat
Chunky Steak & Potato	10¾ oz.	1½ bread, 1½ meat
Chunky Vegetable	10¾ oz.	1 bread, 1 vegetable, 1 fat

CAMPBELL'S LOW SODIUM PRODUCTS (1 CAN, UNDILUTED OZ)

Food Name	Serving Size	Exchange Information
Chicken Noodle	7¼ oz.	1 bread, ½ fat
Chunky Chicken	7¼ oz.	1 bread, 1 meat, ½ fat
Green Pea	7½ oz.	1½ bread, ½ meat, ½ fat
Mushroom, Cream of	7¼ oz.	½ bread, 2 fat
Tomato	7¼ oz.	1 bread, 1 vegetable, 1 fat
Turkey Noodle	7¼ oz.	½ bread, ½ fat
Vegetable	7¼ oz.	1 bread, ½ fat
Vegetable Beef	7¼ oz.	1 vegetable, 1 meat
"V-8" Cocktail Vegetable Juice	6 oz.	1 vegetable

OTHER CAMPBELL'S CANNED PRODUCTS

Food Name	Serving Size	Exchange Information
Barbecue Beans	4 oz.	1½ bread, ½ fat
Home Style Beans	4 oz.	1½ bread, ½ fat
Pork & Beans	4 oz.	1½ bread, ½ fat

Food Name	Serving Size	Exchange Information
Tomato Juice	6 oz.	1 vegetable
"V-8" Cocktail Vegetable Juice	6 oz.	1 vegetable
"V-8" Spicy Hot Cocktail Veg. Juice	6 oz.	1 vegetable

CAMPBELL'S PASTA

Food Name	Serving Size	Exchange Information
Macaroni w/Cheese	1 cup	1½ bread, 1 meat
Italian Style Spaghetti	1 cup	2 bread
Spaghetti and Ground Beef	1 cup	1½ bread, 1 meat, 1 fat
Spaghetti and Tomato Sauce	1 cup	2 bread
Spaghetti and Meatballs	1 cup	1½ bread, 1 meat, 1 fat
Spaghetti Sauce and Meat	1 cup	1 bread, 1 meat, 1 fat
Spaghetti Sauce and Mushrooms	1 cup	1½ bread, 2 fat

CHEF BOY-AR-DEE PRODUCT

Food Name	Serving Size	Exchange Information
Spaghetti Sauce w/Meat	½ can (4 oz.)	1 bread, ½ meat, 1 fat
Spaghetti Sauce w/Mushrooms	½ can (4 oz.)	1 bread, ½ meat, 1 fat
Pizza Sauce	2 oz.	1 fat
Mushrooms in Brown Gravy	5 oz.	1 vegetable, 1 fat
Beefaroni	⅓ can (5 oz.)	1 bread, 1 meat
Cheese Ravioli	⅓ can (5 oz.)	1½ bread, ½ meat, 1 fat
Chili Con Carne w/Beans	⅓ can (5 oz.)	1½ bread, 1 fat

Food Name	Serving Size	Exchange Information
Marinara Sauce	½ cup	1 bread
Meatballs w/Gravy	⅓ can (5 oz.)	½ bread, 2 meat, 1 fat
Ravioli w/Beef	⅓ can (5 oz.)	1½ bread, 1 fat
Spaghetti and Meatballs	⅓ can (5 oz.)	1 bread, 1 meat
Spaghetti Sauce w/Meat	⅓ can (5 oz.)	1 bread, 1 fat
Spaghetti Sauce w/Meatballs	⅓ can (5 oz.)	1½ bread, 1 meat, 1 fat
Spaghetti Sauce w/Mushrooms	⅓ can (5 oz.)	1 bread, ½ fat
Meatball Stew	¼ can (7 oz.)	1 bread, 1 meat, 1 fat
Lasagna	⅕ can (8 oz.)	2 ½ bread, 1 fat
Ravioli w/Beef	⅕ can (8 oz.)	2 ½ bread, 1 fat
Spaghetti & Meatballs	⅕ can (8 oz.)	2 bread, 1 meat, ½ fat
Pizza Pie Mix (made with water)	¼	2 bread, 1 fat
Spaghetti & Meatball Dinner	⅙	3 bread, 1 meat
Spaghetti w/Meat Dinner	⅙	2½ bread, 1 meat
Spaghetti w/Mushroom Dinner	⅙	2 ½ bread
Pizza w/Sausage	⅙	1½ bread, ½ meat, 1 fat
Frozen Beef Ravioli	8 oz.	2½ bread, 1 meat, 1 fat
Frozen Cheese Ravioli	8 oz.	2 bread, 1 meat, 1 fat
Frozen Lasagna	8 oz.	1½ bread, 2 meat, 1 fat
Frozen Manicotti	8 oz.	2 bread, 2 meat, 3 fat

CHUNG KING CORP

Food Name	Serving Size	Exchange Information
Chicken Chow Mein, div.-pak	¼ total mix	2 bread, 2 meat
Beef Chow Mein, div.-pak	¼ total mix	2 bread, 2 meat, 1 fat
Mushroom Chow Mein, div.-pak	¼ total mix	2 bread
Meatless Chow Mein	½ can	1 bread
Subgum Chicken Chow Mein	½ can	1 bread
Beef Chop Suey	½ can	1 bread
Chinese Vegetables	½ can	Free Food
Chop Suey Vegetables	½ can	Free Food
Bean Sprouts	½ can	Free Food
Chow Mein Noodles	½ can	1½ bread, 2 fat
Frozen Chicken Chow Mein	½ pkg. (8 oz.)	1 bread, 1 meat
Soya Sauce		Free Food

GOLDEN GRAIN CO

Food Name	Serving Size	Exchange Information
Spaghetti Dinner	1 cup	3 bread, 1 fat
Cheese Rice-A-Roni	1 cup	2½ bread, 1 meat, 1 fat
Spanish Rice-A-Roni	1 cup	2½ bread, 2 fat
Wild Rice-A-Roni	1 cup	3 bread, 2 fat
Twist-A-Roni	1 cup	2½ bread, 1 fat
Scallop-A-Roni	1 cup	2 bread, 1 meat

GREEN GIANT

Food Name	Serving Size	Exchange Information
Broccoli-Cauliflower Medley	½ cup	½ bread, ½ vegetable, ½ fat
Broccoli Fanfare	½ cup	½ bread, 1 vegetable, ½ fat
Cauliflower in Cheese Sauce	½ cup	1 vegetable, ½ fat
Okra Gumbo	½ cup	1 vegetable, 2 fat
Rice and Broccoli	½ cup	1 vegetable, 1 bread, 1 fat
Rice Pilaf	½ cup	1½ bread, ½ fat
White and Wild Rice	½ cup	1½ bread, ½ fat

KRAFT A LA CARTE SINGLE SERVING POUCHES

Food Name	Serving Size	Exchange Information
Beef Stew	one pouch	2 meat, 1½ bread, 2½ fat
Macaroni and Beef	one pouch	2 meat, 1½ bread, 1½ fat
Salisbury Steak	one pouch	2 meat, ½ bread, 1½ fat
Sweet 'n Sour Pork	one pouch	2 meat, 2 bread, 1 fat

KRAFT MIXES

Food Name	Serving Size	Exchange Information
American-style Spaghetti Dinner Mix	1 cup	3 bread, 1 fat
Cheese Pizza Mix	¼ box	1 meat, 2½ bread, 1 fat
Macaroni and Cheese Dinner Mix	1 cup	½ meat, 2½ bread, 1½ fat

MORTON BRAND TV DINNERS

Food Name	Serving Size	Exchange Information
Ham	1 package	1 bread, 5 meat (omit applesauce)

Food Name	Serving Size	Exchange Information
Turkey, Beef, Salisbury Steak, Meatloaf, and Fish	1 package	1 bread, 1 vegetable, 5 meat
Shrimp	1 package	1 bread, 1 veg, 4 meat, 1 fat

RAGU BRAND

Food Name	Serving Size	Exchange Information
Homestyle Spaghetti Sauce	4 oz.	1 bread, ½ fat
Homestyle Spaghetti Sauce with Mushrooms	4 oz.	1 bread, ½ fat
Homestyle Spaghetti Sauce Flavored with Meat	4 oz.	1 bread, ½ fat

SWANSON CANNED PRODUCTS

Food Name	Serving Size	Exchange Information
Chunk Chicken	2½ oz.	2 meat
Chunk White Chicken	2½ oz.	2 meat
Chunk Thigh Chicken	2½ oz.	2 meat
Chunk Style Mixin Chicken	2½ oz.	2 meat, ½ fat
Chunk Turkey	2½ oz.	2 meat
Chicken Spread	1 oz.	½ meat, 1 fat
Beef Broth	7¼ oz.	Free Food (18-calorie serving)
Chicken Broth	7¼ oz.	1 fat
Beef Stew	7⅝ oz.	1 bread, 1 meat, ½ fat
Chicken Stew	7⅝ oz.	1 bread, 1 meat, 1 fat
Chicken a la King	5¼ oz.	½ bread, 1 meat, 2 fat
Chicken and Dumplings	7½ oz.	1 bread, 1 meat, 2 fat

SWANSON FROZEN PRODUCTS (MEAT PIES

Food Name	Serving Size	Exchange Information
Beef	one 8-ounce pie	3 bread, 1 meat, 4 fat
Chicken	one 8-ounce pie	3 bread, 1 meat, 4 fat
Turkey	one 8-ounce pie	3 bread, 1 meat, 4½ fat
Macaroni and Cheese	one 7-ounce pie	2 bread, 1 meat, 1 fat

SWANSON FROZEN HUNGRY-MAN MEAT PIES

Food Name	Serving Size	Exchange Information
Beef	one 16-ounce pie	4 bread, 3 meat, 7 fat, 1 veg
Chicken	one 16-ounce pie	4 bread, 3 meat, 7 fat, 1 veg
Steakburger	one 16-ounce pie	4 bread, 3 meat, 8 fat, 1 veg
Turkey	one 16-ounce pie	4 bread, 3 meat, 7½ fats, 1 veg

SWANSON FROZEN ENTREES (ONE COMPLETE ENTREE, OZ

Food Name	Serving Size	Exchange Information
Chicken Nibbles w/French Fries	5 oz.	2 bread, 1½ meat, 3 fat
Fish 'n Chips	5 oz.	1½ bread, 2 meat, 2 fat
French Toast w/Sausages	4½ oz.	1½ bread, 2 meat, 2 fat
Fried Chicken w/Whipped Potatoes	7¼ oz.	2 bread, 2½ meat, 3 fat
Gravy and Sliced Beef w/ Whipped Potatoes	8 oz.	1 bread, 2 meat, ½ fat
Meatballs w/Brown Gravy and Whipped Potatoes	9¼ oz.	2 bread, 2 meat, 2 fat
Meatloaf w/Tomato Sauce and Whipped Potatoes	9 oz.	2 bread, 2 meat, 2 fat

Food Name	Serving Size	Exchange Information
Omelets w/Cheese Sauce & Ham	8 oz.	1 bread, 2½ meat, 4 fat
Pancakes and Sausages	6 oz.	3 bread, 1 meat, 5 fat
Salisbury Steak w/Crinkle-cut Potatoes	5½ oz.	2 bread, 1½ meat, 3 fat
Scrambled Eggs and Sausage w/ Hash Brown Potatoes	6¼ oz.	1½ bread, 2 meat, 5 fat
Spaghetti with Breaded Veal	8¼ oz.	1½ bread, 1 meat, 2 fat, 1 veg
Spanish Style Omelet	8 oz.	1 bread, 1 meat, 3 fat
Turkey/Gravy/Dressing w/ Whipped Potatoes	8¾ oz.	1½ bread, 2 meat, 1 fat

SWANSON HUNGRY MAN ENTREES

Food Name	Serving Size	Exchange Information
Barbecue Flavored Chicken w/Whipped Potatoes	12 oz. **	3 bread, 4 meat, 3 fat
Fried Chicken w/Whipped Potatoes	12 oz. **	2½ bread, 5 meat, 4 fat
Fried Chicken Breast Portions	11¾ oz. **	3 bread, 6 meat, 4 fat
Fried Chicken Drumsticks	10¾ oz. **	2½ bread, 4 meat, 5 fat
Lasagna and Garlic Roll	12¾ oz.	3 bread, 2 meat, 5 fat
Salisbury Steak w/Crinkle-Cut Potatoes	12½ oz.	2½ bread, 4 meat, 5½ fat
Sliced Beef w/Whipped Potatoes	12¼ oz.	1½ bread, 4 meat
Turkey/Gravy/Dressing w/ Whipped Potatoes	13¼ oz.	2 bread, 4 meat, ½ fat

*** Edible Portion*

Swanson Frozen Main Course (One Complete Entree, Oz

Food Name	Serving Size	Exchange Information
Chicken Cacciatore	11½ oz.	½ bread, 4 meat, 1 vegetable
Chicken in White Wine Sauce	8¼ oz.	1 bread, 3 meat, 3 fat
Creamed Chipped Beef	10½ oz.	1 bread, 2 meat, 3½ fat
Filet of Haddock Almondine	7½ oz.	½ bread, 4 meat, 2½ fat
Lasagna w/Meat in Tomato Sauce	12¼ oz.	3½ bread, 2 meat, 3 fat
Macaroni and Cheese	12 oz.	2½ bread, 2 meat, 3 fat
Salisbury Steak w/Gravy	10 oz.	1 bread, 3½ meat, 3½ fat
Steak and Green Peppers in Oriental Style Sauce	8½ oz.	½ bread, 2½ meat, 1 vegetable
Turkey w/Gravy and Dressing	9¼ oz.	1½ bread, 4 meat

Lean Cuisine

Food Name	Exchange Information
Breast of Chicken in Herb Cream Sauce	2½ meat, ½ bread, ½ veg, ½ milk
Breast of Chicken Marsala w/Vegetables	2½ meat, ½ bread, 1 veg
Breast of Chicken Parmesan	2½ meat, 1 bread, 1 veg
Cheese Cannelloni w/Tomato Sauce	2 meat, 1 bread, 1 veg
Chicken a L'orange w/Almond Rice	2 meat, 2 bread
Chicken & Vegetables w/Vermicelli	2 meat, 1½ bread, 1 veg, ½ fat
Chicken Cacciatore w/Vermicelli	2½ meat, 1 bread, 2 veg
Chicken Chow Mein w/Rice	1 meat, 2 bread, 1 veg
Chicken Oriental	2 meat, 1½ bread, ½ veg

Food Name	Exchange Information
Filet of Fish Divan	3 meat, ½ bread, ½ veg, ½ milk
Filet of Fish Florentine	3 meat, 1 veg, ½ milk
Filet of Fish Jardiniere & Souffled Potatoes	3 meat, ½ bread, 1 veg, ½ milk
Glazed Chicken w/Vegetable Rice	3 meat, 1½ bread
Lasagna w/Meat Sauce	2½ meat, 1½ bread, ½ veg
Linguini w/Clam Sauce	1½ meat, 2 bread, ½ fat
Meatball Stew	2½ meat, 1 bread, ½ veg, ½ fat
Oriental Beef w/Vegetables & Rice	2 meat, 1½ bread, ½ veg
Rigatoni Bake w/Meat Sauce & Cheese	2 meat, 1 bread, 1½ veg
Salisbury Steak, Italian sauce, vegetables	3 meat, ½ bread, 1 veg, 1 fat
Shrimp & Chicken Cantonese w/Noodles	2½ meat, 1 bread, 1 veg, ½ fat
Sliced Turkey Breast w/Mushroom Sauce	2 meat, 1 bread, ½ veg, ½ milk
Spaghetti w/Beef & Mushroom Sauce	1 meat, 2 bread, 1½ veg
Stuffed Cabbage w/Meat & Tomato Sauce	1½ meat, ½ bread, 2 veg, ½ fat
Szechwan Beef w/Noodles & vegetables	2 meat, 1½ bread, ½ veg, ½ fat
Turkey Dijon	2½ meat, ½ bread, 1 veg, ½ milk, ½ fat
Veal Primavera	2½ meat, 1 bread, ½ veg, ½ fat
Vegetables & Pasta Mornay w/Ham	1 meat, 1 bread, 1 veg, ½ milk, 1 fat
Zucchini Lasagna	2 meat, 1½ bread, 1 veg

WEIGHT WATCHERS FROZEN ENTREES

Food Name	Exchange Information
Chicken Fettucini	2 meat, 1½ bread, 1 fat, ¼ milk
Stuffed Turkey Breast	2 meat, ½ bread, 1 fat, 1½ veg
Southern Fried Chicken Patty	3 meat, 1 bread, ½ veg, 2 fat
Chicken Nuggets	2 meat, ½ bread, 1 fat
Chicken Patty Parmigiana	3 meat, ½ bread, 1 fat, 1½ veg
Imperial Chicken	2 meat, 1 bread, 1 veg, ½ fat
Chicken a la King	2 meat, ½ bread, ½ veg, 1 fat, ½ milk
Sweet 'n Sour Chicken Tenders	1½ meat, 1 bread, 1 veg, 1 fruit
Beef Salisbury Steak Romana	2½ meat, 1 bread, 1 veg, 1 fat
Chopped Beef Steak	3 meat, 1 veg
Veal Patty Parmigiana	3 meat, 1½ veg
Beef Stroganoff	2 meat, 1 bread, ½ veg, 1 fat, ¼ milk
Filet of Fish Au Gratin	3½ meat, ½ bread, 1 veg
Oven Fried Fish	3 meat, ½ bread, ½ veg, 2 fat
Stuffed Sole w/Newburg Sauce	2½ meat, 1 bread, ½ veg, 1 fat, ½ milk
Seafood Linguini	1½ meat, 1 bread, ½ veg, 1 fat
Broccoli & Cheese Baked Potato	1 meat, 1½ bread, 1 veg, ¼ milk
Chicken Divan Baked Potato	1½ meat, 1½ bread, ½ veg, ¼ milk
Pasta Primavera	1 meat, 1 bread, 1 veg, ½ fat, ¼ milk
Lasagna w/Meat Sauce	2 meat, 1 bread, 1 veg, ½ fat
Italian Cheese Lasagna	2 meat, 1 bread, 1 veg, ½ fat
Pasta Rigati	2 meat, 1 bread, 1 veg,
Baked Cheese Ravioli	2 meat, 1 bread, 1 veg,
Spaghetti w/Meat Sauce	1½ meat, 1½ bread, 1 veg, ½ fat
Cheese Manicotti	2 meat, 1 bread, 1 veg, ½ fat
Chicken Fajitas	1½ meat, 1½ bread, 1 veg

Food Name	Exchange Information
Beef Fajitas	1½ meat, 1½ bread, 1 veg
Chicken Enchiladas Suiza	2 meat, 1 bread, ½ veg, ¼ milk
Beef Enchiladas Ranchero	2 meat, 1 bread, 1 veg
Cheese Enchiladas Ranchero	2 meat, 1 bread, 1 veg
Beefsteak Burrito	1½ meat, 1½ bread, 1 veg, ½ fat
Chicken Burrito	1½ meat, 1½ bread, 1 veg, 1 fat
Deluxe Combination Pizza	1½ meat, 1½ bread, ½ veg
Sausage Pizza	2 meat, 1½ bread, ¼ veg
Pepperoni Pizza	1½ meat, 1½ bread, ¼ veg
Cheese Pizza	2 meat, 2 bread, ¼ veg
Pepperoni French Bread Pizza	1½ meat, 2 bread, 1 fat, ½ veg
Cheese French Bread Pizza	1½ meat, 2 bread, 1 fat, ½ veg
Deluxe French Bread Pizza	1½ meat, 2 bread, ½ fat, ½ veg

CAFE CLASSICS (ONE COMPLETE ENTREE, OZ.)

Food Name	Serv. Size	Exchange Information
Baked Chicken	8⅝	1½ meat, 2 bread
Baked Fish	9	1½ meat, 2 bread, ¼ milk, ½ fat
Beef Peppercorn	8¾	1½ meat, 1½ bread, 1 veg, ¼ milk
Beef Portabello	9	2 meat, 1 bread, 1 veg
Beef Pot Roast	9	1½ meat, 1 bread, 1 veg
Bow Tie Pasta & Chicken	9½	1 meat, 2 bread, 1 veg
Cheese Lasagna w/Chicken	10	2 meat, 1½ bread, 1½ veg
Chicken a L'Orange	9	2 meat, 2 bread, ½ veg
Chicken and Vegetables	10½	1½ meat, 1½ bread, 1½ veg
Chicken Carbonara	9	1½ meat, 1½ bread, ½ veg, ½ milk
Chicken in Peanut Sauce	9	1½ meat, 2 bread, ½ veg, ½ milk

Food Name	Serv. Size	Exchange Information
Chicken in Wine Sauce	8⅛	1½ meat, 1½ bread, ½ veg
Chicken Mediterranean	10½	1½ meat, 2 bread, 1 veg
Chicken Parmesan	10⅞	2 meat, 1½ bread, 1½ veg
Chicken Piccata	9	1½ meat, 2 bread, ¼ milk
Chicken w/Basil Cream Sauce	8½	1½ meat, 1½ bread, ½ milk, ½ fat
Chicken w/Almonds	8½	1½ meat, 2½ bread, ½ veg
Fiesta Grilled Chicken	8½	1½ meat, 2 bread, 1 veg
Glazed Chicken	8½	2 meat, 1½ bread, ½ veg
Glazed Turkey Tenderloins	9	1½ meat, 2 bread, ½ milk
Grilled Chicken	9⅜	1½ meat, 1½ bread, ½ veg, ½ milk
Herb Roasted Chicken	8	2 meat, 1 bread, 1 veg
Honey Mustard Chicken	8	1½ meat, 1½ bread, ½ milk
Honey Roasted Chicken	8½	1½ meat, 2½ bread
Honey Roasted Pork	9½	2 meat, 1½ bread, ½ veg
Meatloaf & Whipped Potatoes	9⅜	2 meat, 1½ bread, 1 veg
Orange Beef	9	1½ meat, 3 bread
Oriental Beef	9¼	1½ meat, 1½ bread, 1 veg
Oven Roasted Beef	9¼	1½ meat, 1 bread, ½ veg, ½ milk, ½ fat
Roasted Garlic Chicken	8½	1½ meat, 1½ bread, ½ veg
Roasted Turkey Breast	9¾	1½ meat, 1 bread, 2 fruit
Salisbury Steak	9½	2½ meat, 1½ bread, ¼ milk
Sesame Chicken	9	1½ meat, 3 bread, ½ fruit, ½ fat
Shrimp & Angel Hair Pasta	10	1 meat, 2 bread, ½ veg, ½ milk, ½ fat
Southern Beef Tips	8¾	1½ meat, 2½ bread, 1 veg

Food Name	Serv. Size	Exchange Information
Sweet+Sour Chicken	10	1½ meat, 2 bread, 1 veg, ½ fruit
Teriyaki Chicken	10	1½ meat, 2½ bread
Thai-Style Chicken	9	1½ meat, 2 bread, ½ veg
Chicken Fried Rice Bowl	12	1½ meat, 1 bread, 1 veg
Chicken Teriyaki Bowl	11½	1½ meat, 2½ bread, 1 veg
Creamy Chicken & Veg. Bowl	12	2 meat, 2½ bread, 1 veg, ½ milk
Grilled Chicken Caesar Bowl	10	1½ meat, 2 bread, 1 veg, ½ fat
Teriyaki Steak Bowl	12	1½ meat, 3 bread, 1 veg, ½ fat
3-Cheese Stuffed Rig. Bowl	11⅜	1½ meat, 2 bread, 2 veg

EVERYDAY FAVORITES (ONE COMPLETE ENTREE, OZ.)

Food Name	Serv. Size	Exchange Information
Alfredo Pasta Primavera	10	2 bread, 1 veg, ½ milk, 1½ fat
Angel Hair Pasta	10	2 bread, 2 veg, ½ fat
Baked Chicken Florentine	8	1 meat, 1½ bread, ½ veg, ¼ milk
Cheese Cannelloni	9⅛	1½ meat, 1½ bread, 1 veg
Cheese Lasagna	10	1 meat, 1½ bread, 2 veg, ½ fat
Cheese Ravioli	8½	1 fat, 2 bread, 1 veg
Chicken Chow Mein	9	1 meat, 2 bread, ½ veg
Chicken Enchilada	9	1 meat, 2 bread, ½ veg, ½ milk
Chicken Fettucini	9½	2 meat, 2 bread, ¼ skim milk
Chicken Florentine Lasagna	10	1½ meat, 1½ bread, ½ veg, ½ milk

114

Food Name	Serv. Size	Exchange Information
Classic Five Cheese Lasagna	11½	1½ meat, 2½ bread, 1½ veg, ½ fat
Deluxe Cheddar Potato	10⅜	1 meat, 1½ bread, 1 veg, ½ milk
Fettucini Alfredo	9¼	2½ bread, ½ milk, 1 fat
Hunan Beef & Broccoli	8½	1 meat, 2 bread, ½ veg
Lasagna w/Meat Sauce	10½	1½ meat, 2 bread, 1½ veg, ½ fat
Macaroni and Beef	9½	1 meat, 2 bread, 1 vegetable
Macaroni and Cheese	10	½ meat, 2½ bread, ½ milk
Mandarin Chicken	9	1½ meat, 2 bread, 1 veg
Oriental Style Pot Stickers	9	1 meat, 3½ bread, ½ veg
Penne Pasta w/Tomato	10	2½ bread, 2 veg, ½ fat
Roasted Chicken	8⅛	1½ meat, 2 bread, ½ veg
Roasted Potatoes w/Broccoli	10¼	½ meat, 1½ bread, 1 veg, ½ milk
Santa Fe Rice & Beans	10⅜	2½ bread, 1½ veg, ½ milk, ½ fat
Spaghetti w/Meat Sauce	11½	1 meat, 2½ bread, 1½ veg
Spaghetti w/Meatballs	9½	1 meat, 2 bread, 1 veg, ½ fat
Stuffed Cabbage	9½	1 meat, 1 bread, 1 veg, ½ fat
Swedish Meatballs	9⅛	2 meat, 2 bread
Teriyaki Stir-Fry	10	1½ meat, 2½ bread, ½ veg
Three Bean Chili	10	1 meat, 2 bread, 2 veg
Vegetable Eggroll	9	3½ bread, 1 vegetable, 1 fat
French Bread Pizza Cheese	6	1½ meat, 3 bread, 1 veg
French Bread Pizza Deluxe	6⅛	1½ fat, 2½ bread, ½ veg
French Bread Pizza Pepperoni	5¼	1½ fat, 2½ bread, ½ veg

DINNERTIME SELECTIONS (ONE COMPLETE ENTREE, OZ.)

Food Name	Serv. Size	Exchange Information
Beef Steak Tips Dijon	12	1½ meat, 2 bread, 1½ veg, ½ milk
Chicken Fettucini	13⅝	2 meat, 2½ bread, 1 veg, ½ milk, ½ fat
Chicken Florentine	13¼	2 meat, 2 bread, 2 veg, ½ milk
Glazed Chicken	13	2½ meat, 2 bread, 1½ veg, ½ fat
Grilled Chicken & Penne Pasta	14	2 meat, 2 bread, 2 veg, ½ fat
Grilled Chicken Tuscan	12½	1½ meat, 2 bread, 2 veg
Jumbo Rigatoni	15⅜	2 meat, 2½ bread, 2½ veg, ½ fat
Oriental Glazed Chicken	14	2 meat, 2 bread, 2 veg
Roasted Chicken	12½	2 meat, 2½ bread, 1 veg, ½ milk
Roasted Turkey Breast	14	2 meat, 2½ bread, 2 veg
Salisbury Steak	15½	2 meat, 2 bread, 2 veg

SKILLET SENSATIONS (** DENOTES MORE THAN ONE SERVING)

Food Name	Serv. Size	Exchange Information
Beef Teriyaki & Rice	24**	1 meat, 1½ bread, 1 veg
Chicken Alfredo	24**	1 meat, 1 bread, 1 veg, ½ milk
Chicken Oriental	24**	1 meat, 1 bread, 1 vegetable
Chicken Primavera	24**	1 meat, 1½ bread, 1 veg
Chicken Teriyaki	24**	1 meat, 1½ bread, 1 veg
Garlic Chicken	24**	1 meat, 1½ bread, 1 veg
Herb Chicken & Roasted Pot.	24**	1 meat, 1 bread, 1 veg, ½ milk
Roasted Turkey	24**	½ meat, 1½ bread, ½ veg
Three Cheese Chicken	24**	1 meat, 1 bread, 1 veg, ½ milk

Uncle Ben's Pasta Bowls (All Exchanges Are Approximate, But Close Enough.)

Food Name	Serv. Size	Exchange Information
Chicken Fettuccine Alfredo	350 cal	4 bread, 1 meat, 2 fat
Garden Vegetable Lasagna	300 cal	3 bread, 1 veg, 1 fat
Parmesan Shrimp Penne	380 cal	4 bread, 1 meat, 3 fat
Garlic Chicken & bowties	380 cal	4 bread, 2 meat, 2 fat
Three Cheese Ravioli	380 cal	4 bread, 2 meat, 2 fat
Four Cheese Lasagna	330 cal	3 bread, 2 meat, 1 fat
Chili Bowl with beans & rice	360 cal	2 bread, 4 meat, 1 fat

Chef's Recipe — Has a number of bean and rice dishes, with 1 cup cooked of any of them being about 200 calories and equal to three starch portions.

CHAPTER EIGHT

CHANGING YOUR BEHAVIOR... ONCE AND FOR ALL

"We become what we repeatedly do" - Sean Covey

This chapter is one of the most important in the book. Knowing what to eat is a significant skill to learn, as is walking or other ways of exercising each day. But equally important is changing your behavior and your thinking.

You must stop thinking like a fat person, and start thinking like a thin person.

That's hard, you say? Certainly it's hard.

How do I know?

Because I was fat once; very fat. And I thought like a fat person. So I know, firsthand, that you can change your thinking, and that you can lose weight and keep it off for the rest of your life.

I was a fat medical student, who became an even fatter physician. In 1967, my top weight was slightly more than 240 pounds (I'm six feet tall), in spite of repeated attempts to diet and lose the excess pounds that I knew were shortening my life.

I finally went on a "diet." By the end of 1967, I had reached a goal weight of 180 and resolved never again to let my obesity, and "fat thinking," get the best of me.

Guess what happened? You know all too well. I put the weight back on. Do you know why? Because I had lost my weight on sheer nerve and fear of dying at too early an age. I had not really changed my thought patterns, my fat thinking.

The following story illustrates what I'm trying to say.

I was in Charlotte, N.C., on a business trip. My plane was to leave there about 7 p.m., but the Atlanta airport was fogged in and all incoming traffic was diverted. The airline provided a direct bus for the passengers trying to get to Atlanta, and I decided to take their offer and travel the four hours by bus, instead of waiting to fly out of Charlotte the next morning.

There was no time to get a proper dinner at the Charlotte airport, and I did not realize that the airline had provided a lunch for each passenger.

Something in me seemed to panic. I had to get something to eat! I would be out of reach of food for hours and I hadn't had any supper!

The child in me came out. The next thing I knew, I was standing in the line to get on the bus with four sandwiches, two cartons of milk, several packs of crackers, and a candy bar in my hand.

Common sense should have told me that any adult can delay eating for as long as a day, without suffering any harmful effects. A four or five hour delay in getting my evening meal wouldn't hurt me, but the fear of not eating was still rooted deeply within my mind.

I look back on that episode as my first awakening to my real problem. I was still thinking like a fat man, in spite of my newly found slimness. It's funny now, but it wasn't so pleasant at the time. As you might gather, I survived the trip to Atlanta on the bus.

Right then, I resolved to take a good look inside my own mind and see how the flaw in my thinking processes affected me in everyday life. The information I gained from taking that look, plus the behavior-changing information and hints in this chapter, should help you to see your own self a little more clearly. Self-knowledge is a powerful tool when used wisely.

COGNITIVE RESTRUCTURING IN SLIMMING

Cognitive restructuring (CR) refers to a process of changing a person's thinking, and his or her responses to a particular situation. Cognitive actually refers to the thinking and reasoning processes. In the case of those trying to lose unwanted fat, the goal is to change fat thinking into slim thinking.

To be effective in changing your thinking, you have to practice. Here's what you do: think out particular conditions and situations then come up with desirable and practical responses. Analyze the consequences of each response and decide whether or not this response is a desirable one, producing the desired results. It's a simple but effective process. For example:

SITUATION: You're out shopping with a friend and she suggests you both go to a restaurant where you know there's NOTHING much you can eat on your weight loss program. In the past, every time you've gone to that restaurant, it's been a disaster and you've pigged out. There are other restaurants in the area that are more conducive to your weight loss program. What do you do?

RESPONSE NUMBER ONE: Go along and try to survive at the problem restaurant.

RESPONSE NUMBER TWO: Tell your friend that you want to have lunch with her, but would rather go to_____(a restaurant with a salad bar and fewer problem foods).

After looking at those two possibilities, you obviously would pick number two. Your friend might be upset or annoyed, but you can practice being persuasive to her many times in your mind before the actual situation occurs. You've already responded to her in your mind many times, making it more likely that you'll act in an assertive manner. That is a good opportunity for you to find out if she is really your friend, or just an acquaintance.

SITUATION: You're in a grocery store doing your weekly shopping. You're following your diet program exactly and have been for some time. You're walking by a food display and a salesperson tries to give you a taste sample of your favorite sweet (cookie, cake, candy, etc.). You see this favorite sweet and smell its aroma. You imagine how good it would taste, and you're sorely tempted. Your child (who should have been left at home) begins to beg, plead, and bully you into tasting the sample, not to mention buying some, too.

RESPONSE NUMBER ONE: Give in, eat the sample, and feel guilty immediately. Begin to feel so guilty that you buy several packages of the sweet, take them home, and pig out.

RESPONSE NUMBER TWO: Politely refuse and rapidly steer your cart to another aisle in the store, telling your child firmly but lovingly that you'll decide what to buy, and feeling proud of yourself for having a strong resolve.

You won't be able to imagine all the situations that could affect you at one sitting, but your continuing experience as you slim will build your list of situations that could threaten your compliance with this program. Here is one more, and then there will be space for you to write some of your own.

SITUATION: You're at a family reunion with a lot of your aunts, grandparents, cousins, and other relatives. The table is literally groaning under the weight of some of your favorite foods, none of which are permitted on the slimming part of your program. Some of these relatives know you've been losing fat, and they pester you to eat, eat, eat. They tell you that you look bad and should not lose any more weight. They even try to shovel food on to your plate when you refuse to go get it yourself.

RESPONSE NUMBER ONE: Give in and hope you can get back on your program when you get away from these pests. Say nothing to them and don't try to fight their attempts to sabotage you. Feel so guilty later that you continue to binge and quit your diet program.

RESPONSE NUMBER TWO: Tell everybody to leave you alone. Get actually unpleasant with each of them. Tell them you want to attend family gatherings, but that you might not in the future if they don't leave you alone.

RESPONSE NUMBER THREE: Bring your own food, including lots of raw and lightly steamed vegetables. Quietly make sure that your plate is FULL of food, but your OWN food. Save up a lot of your daily food allotment for this meal with your relatives. The saving and the bringing of your allotted food require planning, so make up your mind that this is necessary. Scout the food spread that your relatives have laid out on the table. Pick and choose a couple of items that conform to your slimming program. Go back several times, getting a small quantity of one item each time. Eat slowly and stay on your program during the entire social function. If you are urged to eat something that was made "just for you," say that you will as soon as you can. Leave the reunion happier than you would have been because of your success at staying on your routine under pressure.

See? It's not that hard to mentally work things out. Now it's your turn to practice. On the next few pages are some blank CR practice forms. Fill them out, or make new ones of your own. Good luck, both on your mental exercises and in the real thing.

SITUATION:

RESPONSE NUMBER ONE:

RESPONSE NUMBER TWO:

RESPONSE NUMBER THREE:

CONSEQUENCES OF MY CHOICE OF ACTION:

SITUATION:

RESPONSE NUMBER ONE:

RESPONSE NUMBER TWO:

RESPONSE NUMBER THREE:

CONSEQUENCES OF MY CHOICE OF ACTION:

GUILT VERSUS REALISM IN WEIGHT REDUCTION

You're learning a skill when you attempt to change the way you deal with food and problem eating habits. Like the learning of any other skill, there are often mistakes associated with the process.

Too many people are destroyed by their errors and are triggered to go on an eating binge when they've only experienced a single problem. If you were learning math, would you let a few troubles make you quit the course? Of course not! So, why let an episode of problem eating ruin your diet program?

This is a form of what is known as "self-defeating behavior" (SDB), and is quite common in the dieting population.

SDB occurs when a person doesn't have the proper insight into what makes him or her behave in a certain way. Going off a diet program, even a little bit, sets off an orgy of guilt, self-accusation, and self-punishment.

The punishment is usually in the form of quitting slimming efforts altogether, or going on a short binge. The self-abuse with food is followed by even more guilt, feelings of helplessness, and more eating.

The only thing you can do to break the cycle is to be aware of this process of self-defeating behavior, and not let it trigger more bad behavior.

Don't be so hard on yourself. Everybody will slip back. Everybody will make mistakes. Don't let it ruin your whole program, and destroy all the efforts you've put so far into your weight loss.

If you have trouble getting started, don't give up. Keep trying!

Rule number one in conquering SDB is to be realistic about what you're trying to do. Your primary goal isn't to lose weight; it's to change your eating habits. An extra pound of water weight on the scale can throw many of you off your programs for no valid reason at all. Do not let a few pints of temporary water gain ruin all your efforts.

I've seen patients go into hysterics because they thought they put on weight, even though it was temporary water weight. Their clothes should have told them they were doing just fine on the program.

If you find yourself deviating from your slimming program, don't just say: "To hell with it, I might as well just eat all I want today!" Go right back on the program at that very moment. Don't binge.

BEHAVIOR MODIFICATION TECHNIQUES THAT WORK

Our behavior is formed in part by our environment and surroundings. You must understand that, from morning to night, we're all bombarded with food commercials, food advertisings, food consumption, and temptations offered by "feeders" and other saboteurs.

Remember, I told you that to lose weight forever, you must think like a thin person, and change your behavior. Here are several behavior-changing techniques that will help you think thin, and change your bad habits into good ones.

Read through these techniques one at a time. I've numbered them, in case you want to jot down the number of one that is particularly helpful to you, so you can refer to it in the future.

You might even want to cut these pages out, and carry them with you, in a briefcase or purse.

Remember, the following are things thin people do. Do them, and start thinking thin.

1. When you've done well, and are losing fat steadily, reward yourself with a non-food treat. Buy a book you've wanted, get a new and smaller piece of clothing, go to a movie (no popcorn, please!), or have some other treat that doesn't involve eating or drinking. Don't use food as a reward. It's a necessity of life, not a reward.
2. Don't eat or drink while you're driving or riding in a car or other vehicle.
3. Don't eat or drink while watching television, listening to the radio, reading, or listening to music. You should have no distractions when eating.
4. Avoid napping or dozing after a meal. Try to move around, either inside or outside your home. Take a short walk, but don't sit down in that recliner, or stretch out on your bed until bedtime. Keep a record of your exercise for each day, even if it's just a short walk. That makes you think about exercise more and prevents the "couch potato syndrome". If you don't exercise, you must put down "NONE" in your daily diary.
5. Keep all sweets that you like out of your house. Tell your family that they're to keep their sweets elsewhere, unless it's a sweet you cannot stand.
6. If you want something cold and sweet, get some plastic popsicle molds and make popsicles with sugar-free Kool Aid or some other sugar-free drink. Don't keep ice cream, ice milk, or frozen desserts in your home.
7. A bowl or cup of partially frozen orange or grapefruit juice with a tiny amount of
8. gelatin added is sometimes enough to satisfy a sweet tooth. Pour the juice into a cup or bowl. Place in the freezer until it just begins to crystallize. Take it out and stir well. Enjoy! Also, look at some of the recipes for treats in Appendix A.
9. Freeze leftovers or discard them. Problem foods that enter your house should never be saved. Use the good and healthy leftover foods later,

but don't eat them now.

10. Use a distinctive placemat whenever you eat. Use a knife, spoon, and fork to eat whatever you're consuming, even if it is, heaven forbid, a candy bar. Set the table, put the candy bar on a plate and slowly eat it using your knife, spoon, and fork. Even at three in the morning set your table if you want that Oreo cookie. Now, after all that, do you still want the cookie, or are you feeling a little bit ridiculous?

11. Avoid "finger food" that is picked up in the hand, nibbled on, dipped into something, or simply is one bite per morsel. This type of food is deadly to a diet. You can consume an enormous amount of this type of food at a party or reception.

12. Stay away from most alcohol during the initial stages of your diet program. Alcohol may slow down your ability to burn fat, speed up your ability to produce fatty tissue, and decrease your inhibitions and sense of control over your eating. It's no accident that the words "Bon Appetit" are spoken as a pre-dinner, alcoholic beverage is consumed.

13. Observe overweight people in restaurants and cafeterias. Be critical, as if you were a dietitian or physician monitoring them. Do they shovel and pour the food in? Is this how you might look? Think about that the next time YOU are eating out.

14. Use a tiny cocktail fork to eat with. Cut your meat and other foods into tinier bites. Eat slowly and see if you aren't eating less. Chopsticks are another way to slow down your eating.

15. Eat soup or salad before every lunch and dinner meal. Eat slowly, using a teaspoon for the soup and a cocktail fork for the salad. Try to make both last twice as long as the previous time you ate them. There does seem to be a delay factor of about 20 minutes from the time eating starts until the brain "knows" it's satisfied. So take your time and give the signals a chance to travel from your stomach to your brain, to tell your brain that your stomach is full.

16. Use a small salad plate instead of a regular-sized dinner plate and see if the same size portion doesn't look larger; put even smaller portions on the smaller salad plate. Visual signals are powerful ones for the obese, both to turn on and turn off eating at certain times.

17. If you're invited to a party, call your hostess up and explain that you're having problems with certain foods. Say the foods don't agree with you (they break you out in fat!), and you would like very much to come, but you don't want to hurt her feelings by appearing not to like the food. See if she can suggest something else for you to eat, or maybe you'll be lucky and there will be nothing but "diet food" at the function. Given the opportunity, most hosts are cooperative and helpful. That is also a good exercise in the use of assertiveness; use cognitive restructuring techniques by practicing in your mind a few times before actually

making the call.

18. At a party, arrive late and leave early, if possible. Have something to eat, even if it's just an apple, before you get there. Sit down somewhere far away from the dips, peanuts, chips, and other high-calorie snacks and finger foods. Get yourself a non-caloric drink, sit down, and enjoy the other guests. If it's a buffet, get at the end of the line and get two items. Eat them and then go back and get one with each subsequent trip until the party is over. If you do it correctly, everyone will wonder why you're losing weight when you're "eating so much." You have only given the appearance of eating a lot, but your hostess will be satisfied.

19. Avoid food-related functions at your place of worship. If you must attend, find out whether the food is being served before or after the function. If before, come in late. If after, get out of there as soon as it's polite to do so. Turn down food offered to you, and say it doesn't agree with you.

20. If you're going to a wedding, anniversary, birthday party, or similar function, where it appears you'll have to eat a lot, save up some of your food portions over the three days prior to the function. You may save ahead and build up a food portion balance, but may not "owe" yourself after the fact and promise to cut down the next few days. Those promises are very hard to keep.

21. When the craving for sweets is at its worse, use a portion of fruit. Cut the fruit up with a knife and eat one tiny morsel of it at a time. Feel the texture and taste of the fruit in your mouth. Chew each bite slowly and carefully, letting the taste buds get the full effect of each bite.

22. When you're just about to raid the refrigerator or pantry for something to eat, get out of the house, or at least the kitchen. Take a walk or do some yard work. Find some task to do and tell yourself that you might have some of whatever food you crave, but first you're going to wait 30 minutes before you have it. If you last 30 minutes, go for a full hour. Keep occupying yourself until the impulse goes away or until an actual mealtime or bedtime comes.

23. If you're an incurable "taster" during cooking, try covering your mouth with a surgical mask or a bandanna. Either one will make you aware of how many times that stirring spoon or fork comes up to your mouth with food on it. The spoon or fork will bump against the mask and make you aware of this unconscious tasting and nibbling. Most hardware and building supply stores have those types of masks for use when a workman is sanding or working around dust.

24. Ask your druggist for a two-ounce bottle with a screw cap. Fill it from a large bottle of diet dressing and carry it in your purse, pocket, or briefcase. Take it along with you when you eat out.

25. When eating out, be sure to tell the server what you want. Don't let

yourself be intimidated by the waiter; if you want an entrée without sauce, or with sauce on the side, tell them. If you want something left off the plate, let the waiter know ahead of time. If it's brought anyhow, ask the waiter to take the plate back and remove the offending item. If you let it sit on your plate, you may nibble on it or eat all of it.

26. Get out of your office when your coworkers start bringing out the snacks or the birthday cake and ice cream. Go wish the other person a happy birthday, happy retirement, etc., but don't let anyone hand you a plate of goodies. Put your hands behind you back and smile, and do not offer to accept it.

27. Instead of staying in your office during lunch and eating (and sharing the wrong foods with others), go outside if the weather permits. Take a walk and get away from your work environment for a while.

28. Establish a set routine for meals and permitted snacks. Try to set up a natural body rhythm that will take hunger, exercise, sleep, and other activities into consideration. Let your routine be your support and protection against problem eating.

29. Avoid bars and taverns for a while until you're a lot stronger than you might be now. Try not to drink, but if you do, drink moderately and concentrate on using diluted drinks (½ jigger of spirits in 12 to 16 ounces of mixer; one ounce of dry wine in 12 ounces of soda) or drink light beer from a jigger glass instead of a mug, can or bottle.

30. If you go to a bar, remember to avoid the salty chips, peanuts, and popcorn. Their purpose is to make you thirsty for several more drinks. When on maintenance, always drink alcohol AFTER a meal, never on an empty stomach. Alcohol before dinner tends to make you eat and drink more.

31. You may be out with a group that has ordered a bottle of wine to share. Have a half glass and let it sit there after the first small sip. If you empty your glass, it gets filled again. If you don't empty it, you don't have to refuse refills. Be sure there's some other type of beverage on the table, with water as the preferred drink. You can also turn your wine glass upside down to avoid ANY wine being poured for you.

32. Sugar-free tonic water, club soda, diet drinks, plain water, mineral water, orange juice, grapefruit juice, and tomato juice are usually in a bar or restaurant. Get this type of drink in these places, or at a party. It looks like you're drinking. If it makes you uncomfortable to be seen without something in your hand, those make good alternative choices instead of alcoholic drinks.

33. Try to make breakfast the biggest meal of your day. If you're not used to eating breakfast, start off slowly and add food gradually over a period of a week. You can also go to bed without supper one night. The next morning you WILL eat. Eat like a king at breakfast, like a

squire at lunch, and like a peasant at dinner.

34. Make yourself perform some kind of work to get your food. Don't have someone else get it for you. Get up and get it yourself. If you do get something, only get a little bit of it and leave the kitchen. Researchers have shown that the lack of immediate contact with food, even if it's only in the next room, is enough to slow or stop extra food intake.

35. Try to make sure that, with the exception of foods prepared for the present meal, there are no easily cooked or ready-to-eat foods in the house. If there is a delay in getting the food because of the necessity to prepare or cook it, the chances are that you might lose the urge long before the snack is ready for you.

36. Never eat standing up or lying down.

37. Avoid secret or closet eating. Have someone who is sympathetic and helpful around if you have a strong urge to eat a problem food.

38. Leave the table immediately after you've finished. Don't remain to watch others eat. There's nothing sacred about someone sitting at the table because of another person's slow eating.

39. Have your family clear their own plates directly into the garbage or disposal. Don't let food sit around; you might go back to the table and nibble.

40. Keep your food in opaque containers that are impossible to see into.

41. Never buy goodies for your family; you'll wind up eating a good percentage of what you bring home. Let your family go off without you for treats. Never take your children to a problem food location, such as a pizza parlor, hamburger stand, frozen yogurt store, Mexican restaurant, or candy store.

42. Try to stay out of food ruts. Vary the types of foods you eat and the ways they're cooked. Boredom is one of your worst enemies. Spices add almost no calories to a dish, but make it interesting and tasty.

43. Do a little pre-planning before you go out to eat. Visualize yourself, using cognitive restructuring, at the restaurant. Imagine how you'll order your food and how you'll tell what your preferences are. Refuse desserts for now. You'll have some later on your maintenance program, but it's better to stay away from these highly concentrated sweets until you're a lot stronger in your habit patterns.

44. Skip the bread, butter, rolls, pre-dinner drinks, and other traps. Ask for a glass of mineral water, or some other harmless beverage, and refuse to get any bread out of the basket. If your restaurant is really service-minded, the waiter may actually put bread on your bread plate. A hand held over the plate is an assertive way to say no without offending.

45. A fruit cup for dessert is a good choice, but make sure it's fresh fruit. Fruit canned in heavy syrup, or in any syrup at all, is loaded with sugar.

In fact, the word syrup refers to sugar dissolved in water.

46. Don't be a "couch potato" and sit all the time. Move around and keep your body healthy. Wear athletic clothes and use them.

47. Be realistic about what you can expect to lose every month. Don't be upset about fluctuations in weight as a result of fluid retention or healthy muscle growth. If your activity pattern allows for two or three pounds of fat loss a week, consider yourself lucky. Only in science fiction, or certain diet books, do we find the 10-pounds-a-week stories and claims. It's physically impossible for most of us to lose more than eight to 10 pounds a month. Our bodies just won't let go of much more than that.

48. When you're at the end of your workday and are tired, hungry, angry, anxious, provoked, and perhaps a dozen other things, too, stop for a minute before entering your home. Plan to have something, such as a tuna salad or fruit plate, when you first step in the door. My Super Soup (recipe is in Appendix A) is another good idea for your homecoming snack. Stop for a minute before you enter your home and visualize yourself having a snack at your table with the placemat and the rest of your place setting in front of you. Avoid going by a fast-food restaurant on the way home and getting something to eat. Visualize yourself going straight home while sitting in your office at the end of the day. Avoid impulse buys of problem foods through this technique.

49. Reward yourself with a soothing hot bath when you've had your snack. Luxuriate in the water and let the heat soak into your body, carrying away all the soreness and the muscle spasms in the neck and the upper back. Feel the tension leaving your body as every muscle in your body relaxes. Your body is now relaxed. It doesn't require problem foods to cover up your nervousness or tension. You can now eat what you NEED, rather than what you CRAVED. You can look forward to a good night's sleep and waking up the next morning refreshed and alert. Those mental images can be real to you if you let them. Treat yourself to a hot bath as a reward for a hard day's work.

50. Put some other barriers between you and food. Try to polish your nails when you're hungry. Another tactic is to find something dirty and grubby to do that will make your hands so filthy that you would not eat at that time. I often dig in my flower garden whenever the urge to eat hits me. Perhaps the cellar, basement, or attic needs a good cleaning. Unless you've hidden the Oreo cookies there, you're probably safe.

51. Chew sugar-free gum the whole time you're cooking a meal. You can also nibble on something benign, such as celery. Cut the celery into small chunks. Chew the celery pieces, but chew them well. Make each chunk last at least three or four minutes.

52. Put encouraging messages around the house, particularly in the kitchen,

on the pantry door, on the refrigerator, and at the bathroom mirror. Say whatever you want. Some that I use are listed below: A MINUTE IN THE MOUTH, AN HOUR IN THE STOMACH, AND A LIFETIME ON THE HIPS. A WAIST IS A TERRIBLE THING TO MIND. DO YOU REALLY NEED THAT? BE HONEST NOW!

53. Find a kindred spirit, who is also dieting, and provide support to each other. Speak to this person every day if possible. Try to walk daily with this person. It pays off for both of you in increased fat loss. That mutual support works! Overeaters Anonymous is often a worthwhile source of help for dieters.

54. Avoid negative people. Divorce yourself from those who would hinder your progress through their own problems in dealing with life.

55. Think thin. Visualize yourself as a thin person with a healthy body and boundless energy. See yourself in thin clothes and outfits.

56. Learn to be assertive with others and yourself. Being assertive means letting your needs be known in a non-aggressive way. It doesn't mean that you have to be rude or obnoxious, just firm.

57. Try to get your grocer or delicatessen worker to weigh things for you in three-ounce or four-ounce packages, and separately wrap them. Portion control starts in the store. Use smaller cans, rather than the larger and more wasteful sizes. Buy leaner cuts of meat.

58. Practice delays during a meal. Deliberately place your utensils on the table and relax for a moment. Try to wait a minute or more before starting to eat again. Use those delays to build confidence in your ability to control your environment, rather than having it control you.

59. If you're in a restaurant and have ordered a standard entree that is too much for you to eat, don't hesitate to take it home, rather than just eating another four ounces of filet or other dish. Don't be embarrassed to ask for help from the waiter.

60. Don't expect miracles. It takes hard work to get down to a slim weight and figure. There's no shortcut in the process. Your habits, thinking, eating, and activity pattern must all change, or the entire process is futile. The good news is that it really isn't that hard to do. The whole thing boils down to making a lot of small changes in your life.

61. Look upon this entire program of weight loss as a learning situation. You're learning a skill and you may make mistakes along the way. Don't be punitive with yourself. Be tolerant and forgiving of yourself and others. Expect to have difficulties and be ready for them. When mistakes or problems arise, look upon them as golden opportunities to show what you can do to excel at the task of slimming yourself.

CHAPTER NINE

EXERCISE: HOW IT CAN HELP YOU STAY THIN, HEALTHY, AND HAPPY

"Exercise is like an addiction. Once you're in it, you feel like your body needs it" – Elsa Pataky

What is it that you hope you lose when you go on a diet? The answer is weight, of course, but the weight of what? Each person's overall weight is made up of two components: lean body mass and fat. Lean body mass (LBM) consists of your bones, vital organ tissues, and water. The other component is fat.

Although most people talk about wanting to lose weight, they are really interested in losing fat, and retaining (or building) lean body mass.

You really shouldn't be concerned with your weight at all, but with your fat. After all, it's the excess fat that jeopardizes your health and detracts from your appearance. If you think about it, you've never heard anyone complain that their muscles are too heavy.

It's been clinically proven that if we lose weight without exercising, we lose too high a proportion of LBM, along with the fat. Since it isn't healthy to lose vital muscle or organ tissue over a period of time, this loss of mostly muscle protein must be minimized. If we aren't careful, the muscle loss can be substantial.

While dieting without exercise can cause you to lose a substantial amount of muscle as well as fat, if you exercise properly while dieting, about 90 percent of the weight you lose will be fat.

If you're wondering how it's possible to tell whether a person is losing fat or LBM, the answer lies in weighing the individual under water, using at least two separate measurements.

I'm sure you won't be weighing yourselves under water, but studies with overweight people have proven that you must exercise while slimming to maintain your lean body mass.

The simplest way to measure whether or not you have lost fat is to observe how your clothes fit you. Some people go down in clothes size and are noticeably smaller, without losing any weight at first. Remember, you are trying to lose fat, not weight. The weight loss may lag, but it eventually catches up with the size change. Don't be a scale watcher; that can only lead to failure. Take the long-term view of what is happening in your body.

The maintenance phase of your program is much, much easier if you've established a good exercise plan, by the time you reach your weight goal.

Exercise is like a habit — a good habit instead of a bad one. If you acquire the habit of exercise while losing weight, you'll keep the habit and be able to maintain your weight loss. And that's your goal: to stay thin forever, not just a short time.

Unfortunately, the only form of exercise practiced by some slimmer's is hopping on and off the scale.

You're going to have to exercise if you want to lose fat, not body mass. And you're going to have to exercise if you want to maintain your weight loss. It's that simple.

It's also important that you realize that a slower-than-expected loss, or actual gain, of body weight may indicate a beneficial change in body composition. What I am referring to is the fact that when you diet and exercise together, you might actually GAIN lean body mass.

If you're losing inches like crazy, but the scale isn't budging, don't worry about it; you're losing fat and gaining valuable LBM. Your friends will all assume that you have lost "weight" because of your slimmer look. If they ask you how much you've lost, simply say: "I've gone from a size __ to a size __."

Since I prefer for exercise to be gentle and progressively more difficult, I highly recommend walking as the best form of exercise.

HOW TO WALK?

I don't have to go into too much detail here. You've been walking your whole life, and you know how to do it naturally. However, here are some guidelines:

Start slowly. If you must walk around the block for five minutes to get started, so be it. The important thing is that you get up off the sofa and DO IT! And, that you do it regularly, every day.

The key word is patience. Don't try to be too ambitious and do too much the first few days. The same defect in reasoning that makes an overweight person try to lose weight too fast is a problem here as well. Be realistic about what you can do to start.

If you're used to walking a half-mile a day, then start with that and build up. If you haven't walked over a hundred yards at a time, start with that.

Walking is as close as any exercise to being perfect for slimmers who have not done any exercise for quite some time.

It's easy to do, doesn't cost any money, isn't boring (and can be rather pleasant), and can be done alone or with a friend.

Weather poor outside? Go to a mall and walk inside. Too hot outside? Don't walk at noon, but later at night (during a sunset) or early in the morning.

See how many options you have?

And you don't need fancy clothes, or equipment. However, a good pair of walking shoes is a must. Go to a sporting goods store, spend a little extra money, and be fitted properly.

Don't start off too fast. The important thing is that you do start, and that you do it regularly. That means every day. (If you occasionally miss a day, don't get discouraged. Start right back with walking the next day.)

Once you've walked a few days and feel better and more comfortable with it, you should start picking up the pace. Swing your arms and walk a little faster each day.

Each person has to realistically set an initial goal, and try to meet that goal. The reasonably healthy person should try a stroll of about 20 minutes for the first few days. Increase the pace slowly until you're walking rapidly and you get a feeling of exertion when you're done.

Once you reach that goal, increase the length and distance of your walk.

Work up to walking three or more miles a day, at a pace of 15 to 20 minutes per mile. A good walk of 40 to 45 minutes or even an hour every day will go a long way in keeping your weight steady. And along with weight control, you'll feel better, healthier. It's a great, easy exercise.

I'm often asked how fast people should walk.

At some point, you want to walk so fast that you'd have a little trouble carrying on a normal conversation. You still can talk, but it would be difficult. You're going too fast if you're gasping for breath.

Here's another way to figure out how fast to walk. Think of the following situation: You're out walking in light clothes, and it turns suddenly very chilly; on top of that, you have to go to the bathroom; you're about 20 minutes from home. How fast would you walk to get home? That's how fast you should walk once you've walked for a while.

MORE STRENUOUS EXERCISE

Some of you will enjoy walking so much; you'll want to do more strenuous exercises. That has happened to many of my patients, and I know it will happen to many of you, too.

However, if you never do anything else but walk, you're still doing yourself a world of good. If every one of you walks regularly, you'll be very successful on The Doctors' Clinic-30 Program.

You can start jogging, but I'd recommend talking to friends who jog, or local sports physicians. You want to make sure you're running the right way, on the right surface, and with the right warm-up and stretching exercises.

Below are some other, higher aerobic exercises you can try, in place of jogging.

THE MINITRAMPOLINE

A few years ago, I first saw a minitrampoline demonstrated during a medical seminar.

I didn't even give the person showing the device the courtesy of trying it. In fact, I almost laughed because I thought it was a ridiculous looking thing.

Since that time, I've completely changed my mind. Shortly after that seminar, I read some medical papers on the use of the minitrampoline and its effectiveness for both losing weight, and maintaining weight loss.

I bought a couple minitrampolines to try them out; I put one in my office to show patients, and another in my home.

I think it is a great tool to help you stay in shape and lose weight.

The great thing about the minitrampoline, or rebounder as it's also called, is that it can help you burn calories, tone muscles, and increase your cardiac reserve. And it is used indoors, so no more excuses about not going out in the rain.

While you bounce up and down on the rebounder, you experience a "gravity massage."

At the top of the bounce, you're traveling upward. Just as you stop upward movement, you weigh slightly less than normal. As you fall down to the surface and decelerate, there's a point at which you stop movement. And before you start up on your next bounce, you weigh slightly more than normal.

When a person bounces up and down on the rebounder, an interesting thing takes place. The change in weight, from weighing slightly more to weighing slightly less, produces a work effect on every muscle in your body.

Each muscle is working against gravity, even the tiny muscles in the face and neck. If there is a constantly changing gravity force, the muscles will, over time, tone up. People have achieved some amazing results on rebounders through this "gravity massage".

Secondly, a rebounder has an aerobic effect. Your body will get a good cardiovascular workout on a rebounder, either through bouncing or running in place.

Finally, the rebounder protects your ankles, knees, hips, and overall bone structure from injuries that you could get when running on a hard surface.

Like walking, you must remember to start slowly. Stand on the rebounder surface and lightly bounce on it until you get used to it. Then bounce more vigorously.

After you get comfortable with the bouncing effect, you can begin an exercise routine. I usually recommend running shoes and loose clothing that you might wear outside the house while running. Play some music with a good beat, and find a large clock with a second-hand that you can use to time yourself.

Start with about a minute of simple bouncing. Then run in place for a minute, at about 120 steps a minute or better. Go back to bouncing for another minute, and then stop for the day. Don't try to do more than that on the first day.

Add 30 to 60 seconds of running in place per day, until you reach 20 minutes, then go to twice a day, if possible.

SWIMMING

This is another of my favorite aerobic exercises. You can burn excess calories — a lot of excess calories — while working your heart and lungs, and keeping your body muscles firmed up.

At first, it isn't necessary to swim laps to produce a training effect. Paddling around in the water will build your stamina and bum calories.

If you don't want to begin by swimming laps, paddle around the pool for 25 or 30 minutes, never letting your feet touch the sides or the bottom of the pool. The constant and unrelenting effort to keep afloat by paddling will really help get you in shape for more vigorous swimming later.

The other benefit to swimming is that you're submerged in mostly cool water. When you swim, the heat from your body will be transferred into the cooler water. The amount of heat lost is dependent on your body temperature, the water temperature, and the surface area of your body that's exposed to the cooler water.

Heats, or calories, are lost that way much more easily than through sweating. The greater the difference between your body temperature and the water temperature, the greater the amount of heat, or calories, that is lost.

The calories lost into the pool don't have to be burned by the body through muscular activity. Since you'll be using your muscles a lot, that is an advantage to you and it accelerates your weight loss.

Finally, if you do decide to swim, make sure you're in a safe environment; either with a swimming partner, or in a pool with a lifeguard on duty. NEVER SWIM ALONE!

SKIING INDOORS, WHERE IT'S WARM

One of the most strenuous activities I've ever attempted is cross-country skiing. The rhythmic motion of the legs and arms produced an aerobic exercise unlike anything else I've ever experienced. If I lived in Minnesota or Colorado, this would be one of my favorite activities.

Since I live in Georgia, there is little chance of cross-country skiing for me, but I found something almost as good; something I can do indoors, all year long. I bought a machine that lets me do cross-country skiing — indoors.

It's light enough to carry with me in my car when I'm on the road for several days. It's small enough to fit underneath my bed, or to stand up in my closet. And the particular unit I bought was reasonably priced. Shop around, and you should be able to buy a good unit, also.

HOW MANY CALORIES CAN I BURN?

Finally, if you need it, here's a chart that tells you how many calories are burned in a 30-minute workout. Values are for a 154-pound person. Those who weigh more may expend more calories, and those less than 154 pounds may expend fewer calories. People differ in the way they walk, run, or bike.

Calories expended per 30 minutes	
Badminton	200
Cycling, a mile in 11 minutes	130
Cycling, a mile in 6.4 minutes	210
Dancing, easy and moderate tempo	110
Dancing, aerobic	350
Gymnastics	140
Horseback riding at trot	230
Judo or Karate, katas and workout	400

Calories expended per 30 minutes

Minitrampoline or rebounder, 100 to 120 steps per minute, low jogging	130
Minitramp—higher step	200
Ping pong, singles	140
Rowing machine, moderate pace	150
Running, 11-minute mile	300
Running, 9-minute mile	410
Running, 6-minute mile	525
Skiing, downhill	250
Skiing, cross-country	300
Squash	440
Stair climbing, up, 60 steps/minute	430
Stair climbing, down, same rate	100
Swimming laps, moderate pace	270
Swimming laps, racing speed	330
Tennis, singles	225
Walking, 20-minute mile	130
Walking, 15-minute mile	200

CHAPTER TEN

FEEDERS AND SABOTEURS

"The person who masters himself through self-control
and discipline is truly undefeatable" – The Buddha

I've referred to feeders and saboteurs before in this program. Basically, these are people who unintentionally, or intentionally, want to ruin your weight loss program.

Any person who's even moderately successful in losing unwanted fat will probably run into one or more of these people. If you're aware beforehand of the tactics they use, you'll have more success at fending off their efforts to destroy your weight loss program.

Obesity is a killer disease and you'd think that no rational and compassionate person would attempt to stop an overweight person from losing unwanted fat. Unfortunately, that is not the case. Almost every person who is losing weight has encountered this situation, some more often than others.

There are three types of feeders, each with a slightly different reason for being that way; each one will be covered in detail. This chapter uses feminine pronouns, but male can also be feeders and saboteurs!

A few case histories are recited in this section to illustrate just how deadly these feeders and saboteurs can be.

THE THIN FEEDER

All of us have seen situations where a thin woman cultivates a friendship with a much heavier woman. If the thin feeder is truly thin, the overweight woman makes her look even thinner.

Someone who is 20 pounds over her desired weight looks thinner than a friend who has 50 pounds of extra fat. If this obese friend begins to lose weight and starts to look more attractive, the relationship is threatened and the thinner person feels the competition, either real or imagined.

The usual behavior of the thin feeder is to try to sabotage her friend and think up places to go where the supply of forbidden foods is abundant. If that fails to work — and it will fail if the slimmer has been warned about this happening — the newly slim woman will find herself without this particular "friend."

Carol and Sally were friends and coworkers in an insurance office in Atlanta. Carol was slightly overweight, but had managed to never get more than 15 pounds over her ideal weight. Sally, a recent divorcee, was the mother of three small children and had gained 80 pounds over her desired weight of 120 pounds. She was friendly and a hard worker, and made Carol seem almost anorexic in comparison. The two of them went to lunch every day and often shopped together, too.

Sally came to see me and a physical exam revealed that she had elevated cholesterol and triglycerides, hypertension, and a symptomatic hiatal hernia.

The initial remedy for all those problems was weight reduction, using a fat-controlled diet. Sally could not eat out for a while and had to eat only food that she prepared at home. Sally now had to walk during her lunch hour and had no more time to eat and shop with Carol. She lost at a steady rate of eight pounds a month, reaching a weight of 160 pounds in five months.

She noticed that Carol started bringing sweets to the office and leaving some of Sally's desk, even though she repeatedly asked Carol not to do so.

After two or three binges on sweets, brought on by this subtle type of sabotage, Sally discussed it with me. A study of her food intake diaries showed that her office was the only place where she had dieting problems.

The instigator in each case was Carol. We discussed the problem and decided to use the "parrot technique" where Sally would tell Carol repeatedly that she did not want the food. It worked. The weight loss resumed at its old rate and within another six months Sally was down to her desired weight and placed on a maintenance program.

Her blood pressure, blood fats, and hiatal hernia symptoms were all improved. She felt wonderful, except that she had to make new friends. Carol, her former close friend, and some of the other office workers had virtually ostracized her. They continued to try to fatten her up by offering tempting food, but they refused to include her in their social activities.

Fortunately, Sally was warned of this and had ignored their hostile acts. She'd been made aware of the dynamics of feeder behavior and had accepted the situation.

Sally is now in her second year of maintenance and has a lot of new, slimmer male and female friends. She recognized that she was being used and refuses to be a victim of feeders.

THE OVERWEIGHT FEEDER

A lot of obese women don't like to be seen in public alone. That is particularly true if public eating is involved. If one overweight female is in an ice cream parlor eating a large sundae, it could make her self-conscious.

If five obese ladies are together, eating the same thing, there seems to be a feeling of mutual support. They are "eating buddies" and help bolster each other's courage in violating "diets" that they claim to sometimes follow.

If one of them becomes a success at slimming and starts shedding pounds and inches, the others may attack with food and temptations involving obviously fattening foods and beverages. They may remark that the slimmer is looking sick, wrinkled, or other equally disparaging and discouraging comments.

Whatever the statement, it's always followed by an invitation, a request, or even a virtual order to eat "just a little bit" of whatever is most fattening.

The overweight feeder is afraid of losing an "eating buddy" and is also quite jealous. A shark or wolverine has more compassion than a feeder, as the next story will illustrate.

Elaine was a teacher at a local elementary school. She became my patient, and an initial exam showed her weight at 300 pounds. She developed problems with her back that caused her extreme pain and disability. It was obvious that she had no choice but to get her weight down as quickly as possible.

She was placed on a sensible weight loss program and watched closely. Weight loss was a predictable and easy two to three pounds a week, with no problems with electrolytes or hunger.

Elaine was previously part of a group of six unmarried or divorced teachers, who were all significantly overweight. One of the six, Hannah, had less fat to lose, and she started a weight loss program the same time as Elaine.

By the time Elaine had lost the first 50 pounds, Hannah had dropped out in response to the pleas of the other four in the group. The usual method of sabotage was to place unwanted and unrequested plates of sweets, or concentrated calories of some other type, in front of Hannah and Elaine. The feeder would then implore both of them to eat something "since it was fixed just for you."

Elaine refused to be the victim of these food bullies, but Hannah was not able to assertively refuse and eventually got discouraged. She resumed her old eating habits, and rapidly regained all of her weight, plus 15 pounds.

The others in the group, including Hannah, now concentrated on Elaine. She was told that she was getting ugly and wrinkled, and that she had really gotten "stuck up" since she lost that weight.

Although she still needed to lose more than a hundred pounds, she was told she didn't need to lose any more weight. Her temperament and disposition were attacked as being terrible and other uncomplimentary things were said about her.

Elaine was instructed early on about the tactics of feeders and was unmoved by all the increasingly disagreeable remarks. She continued to lose weight and got enough confidence in her own abilities to resume her post-graduate studies.

Her increased self-esteem helped her overcome what could have been an overwhelming negative influence on her efforts. She is now principal of another school and has also found herself attractive and slim enough to date several eligible men.

Unfortunately, her five former friends are still part of a gang of overeaters, none of whom has been able to break away from the others and get rid of their unwanted pounds.

The almost malignant influences of the thin feeder and the fat feeder are difficult to combat, but neither type is as deadly and as hard to fight as the next feeder.

THE GRANDPARENT FEEDER

This type of person may not actually be a grandparent and may not even be old, but the archetype is the granny figure with a plate of brownies or some other equally diet-destroying food.

"Now Sonnie (or Missie), you KNOW that this little bit of food can't possibly hurt you. This diet business is silly. Besides, this isn't unhealthy; I made it with pure cream. You're not going to break your poor granny's heart and not have some? I made them just because I knew you were coming to see me."

It would be almost a sin to refuse this kind of plea, particularly since you know that love motivated her, not jealousy or envy.

This type of feeder feels that love is shown best by feeding. Any attempt to reject the offered food is considered a rejection of the grandparent feeder's love, a difficult thing to spurn.

Most slimmer's find that frequent telephone calls to this type of feeder are the best way to maintain contact. The grandmother figure is hard to deal with in person. It's also impossible to convince her that you're right in losing your attractive baby fat, even if you are the parent of grown children yourself.

Take my advice and love her (or him) from a distance. Give her your phone number, but not your address. Otherwise, she'll mail you sweets and fattening foods.

All those examples should make you more observant of your own surroundings. It would benefit each person on this program to observe their environment for seven consecutive days.

List everyone who even remotely offers you food or beverages during that time. List people who made you eat, even if they triggered you to eat through annoyance or some other emotion, and didn't actually offer food.

Try to figure out the tactics of each one and discover a way to overcome their influence. Work out your own methods of dealing with each one and practice these mentally before you actually encounter the person again.

Use the cognitive restructuring you learned about earlier. Your new, thinner life will be much less complicated, not to mention more pleasant and healthy.

CONVERTING FROM HIGH FAT TO LOWER FAT COOKING

Try to Avoid	Healthier options
High Fat Meats	Lean meats such as round, sirloin, chuck arm pot roast, loin, lean, and extra lean ground beef.
Neck bone	Skinless chicken thighs
Ham hocks and fat back	Turkey thighs
Lard, butter, or other fats that	Cook with nonstick pans using small are hard at room temperature amounts of vegetable or olive oil or vegetable sprays.
Pork bacon	Turkey bacon, lean ham, Canadian bacon (omit if on a low sodium diet)
Pork sausage,	Ground skinless turkey ground beef or pork breast or lean chicken sausage
Whole milk	Low fat (1%-2%) or nonfat/skim milk
Whole milk cheeses	Low fat or part skim milk cheeses
Cream	Evaporated skim milk

Try to Avoid	Healthier options
Regular mayonnaise in	Mustard, low fat mayonnaise, salads and sandwiches nonfat yogurt, or low fat salad dressings.
Avocado, olives, eggs,	Fruits and brightly colored etc. as salad garnishes vegetables, and cooked egg whites
Regular bouillon or broth	Low sodium bouillon and broth
Browning and sautéing w/butter	Chicken or beef broth
Deep fat frying, basting with fat,	Broiling, steaming, roasting, baking, cooking in fatty sauces microwaving, grilling, broiling, stewing simmering, stir-frying with a little oil

AN OPEN LETTER TO THE SPOUSE (OR PARENT, OR FRIEND) OF A SLIMMER

(To the reader: Once you've finished reading this section, please give it to your husband, or wife, or father, or mother, or sister, or friend, etc.)

You may think this is a rather unconventional thing to do, appealing to someone close to a slimmer for help, but certain things need to be said, or all the slimmer's efforts will possibly be for nothing.

It's obvious that no one holds an overweight person down and makes him or her overeat. In 99 percent of the cases, overweight people are that way because they eat more food (and calories) than they burn off.

What is not so obvious is the effect that the environment has on overweight people. Numerous scientific experiments have pointed out, time and time again, that the surroundings and external influences on fat people have more to do with their problem eating behavior than the internal cues of hunger.

Most overweight people never experience a true feeling of hunger or of satiety (lack of hunger) in the way that a person of normal weight does. Certain experiments have shown that cues, such as elapsed time from the most recent meal, odors, sight of food (watching TV and eating), being in a certain location, and emotional upset will trigger massive food intake. These cues can make even the most compliant slimmer vulnerable to problem eating.

You may be asking yourself, "What does all this have to do with me? It's not my problem. He (or she) should be able to diet by willpower alone! Why involve me at all? If she (or he) does not do well, the overeating isn't my fault."

Nothing could be further from the truth.

You're important, in fact, more important than most of the people in this slimmer's life, or you wouldn't be reading this now. If you are truly interested in helping the slimmer, please take what is said here on faith for a while and see for yourself whether or not it's true.

It may mean changing your own lifestyle a bit, but the results will be worthwhile.

Here's how you can help:

To begin with, never criticize the slimmer for not slimming properly, or for his or her eating habits. Ridicule, teasing, taunting, or other verbal abuse does not stop undesirable behavior.

All you'll accomplish by doing that is make your loved one or friend eat more than before. You may have to bite your tongue, but only comment on desirable eating behavior. If your loved one or friend is not breaking the diet, then comment on how good that behavior is. If a lapse does occur (and it will), the less said the better. In the long run, positive reinforcement techniques work better than ridicule or intimidation. To repeat, even if you see something done incorrectly, please say nothing.

Since visual or odor cues are important in producing undesirable eating behavior, the slimmer needs to "fat-proof" his or her dwelling. That means all junk food must be cleaned out.

For the rest of your family or social group, it might mean going out to get ice cream. To eat such goodies in front of someone on a diet is the height of cruelty.

Many families are used to eating together, but the slimmer may decide not to eat with you if he or she gets distressed by sitting and watching others eat. He or she may simply eat quickly and then get right up from the table after finishing, even if others have not yet stopped eating.

Many slimmers are pickers, and if such a person remains at the table, it'll be difficult not to nibble at one thing or another. Please be understanding, and at a later date, when slimming efforts have been successful, normal table behavior may be resumed.

A slimmer may have to stay away from problem places, such as pizza parlors, taco stands, spaghetti houses, hamburger stands, take-out fried chicken stores, doughnut parlors, and other equally tempting dens of obesity. Please do not bring this type of food home and tempt the slimmer. The result is usually disastrous and is equivalent to tempting an alcoholic to go into a bar, or to bringing him or her a bottle of whiskey.

No thinking and caring person would do that to an alcoholic, but lots of people will try to "feed" a slimmer.

What this message boils down to is that the slimmer is weak and does have some bad habits, but he or she is worth any and all efforts to help save him or her from the life-shortening effects of obesity.

You and others may be inconvenienced a little, but surely you can tolerate these minor annoyances for a while.

About one of every hundred slimmer's is faced with open or hidden sadism, or mental illness, on the part of his or her spouse or a relative.

A certain type of person seems to feed on the misery of others, particularly of those who are overweight. One example is the husband who keeps his wife fat, usually because of insecurity or other related reasons.

He feels secure because she is so obese that no one else would have her. When his wife tries to lose weight, such a man becomes anxious and tries to get her to go off the diet by tempting her, annoying her, or by sabotaging her efforts. As she gets closer to her lower weight goal, he becomes more and more anxious and may resort to physical abuse, verbal assaults and, as a last desperate effort, may cut off her funds so that she cannot continue her weight loss program.

For those who stick it out and continue the diet program, there is sometimes divorce, usually coming on the heels of an increasing amount of verbal and physical abuse.

Not all victims are wives. Many are husbands of insecure wives, or children of insecure parents. Some men are victims of a bullying, feeding wife. Those women try to get and keep what they want, a husband so fat and unattractive that no one else would want him.

In summary, you and others who have close contact with the slimmer have more influence on him or her than you could ever realize. Without your total assistance and support, the slimmer will more than likely fail.

The attitude that "food is love" is widespread. The idea is still strong in many people that by giving food you show love, and by rejecting that food you also reject that love. You can, however, show love in ways not related to food.

Try flowers and small, inedible gifts to show affection and love. They work just as well and last a lot longer!

CHAPTER ELEVEN

OBESITY, WEIGHTLOSS, AND SEXUAL ACTIVITY

Monogamous, sex between two adult partners is a normal part of living and is healthy and satisfying for all concerned. The significantly obese man or woman should be able to enjoy healthy sex as well as anyone else, but many don't for one reason or another. This book is not a sex manual, but the subject needs addressing because of the many dysfunctional problems that can occur in a man or women with obesity and related problems.

The bad news is that erectile dysfunction (ED) is fairly common in older and/or obese men, and a lack of libido or orgasm is also common in many obese women. The good news is that we have learned a lot about how both male and female sexual dysfunction can be corrected, or at least helped some, by using a little common sense and the services of an understanding and sympathetic physician.

Unless there has been some anatomical destruction of the tissues, nerve supply, or circulation to the male sex apparatus, we can many times improve conditions. With the advent of Viagra, we've solved many problems connected with ED, but even Viagra can't help some of the problems mentioned here that can cause ED or other problems.

Mechanical problems that impede or impair sexual intercourse are often a result of the abdominal obesity pattern (apple shape) that may be present in one or both partners. Not only is it more difficult to have intercourse with all the layers of fat between the two partners, but the energy necessary to perform the sex act may be lacking because the man is in such poor physical shape.

I tell my obese patients to start some sort of walking program or similar exercise in order to build up their aerobic potential. The greater their exercise tolerance, the better they are able to hold up under the demands of sex. Not only do they feel better and perform better, they get thinner in the process, and that could help any existing hypertension, back problems, diabetes, and other obesity-related problems.

A drop of only 10 to 20% of body weight can markedly reduce many elevated blood pressures to a more normal level. That might mean any blood pressure medication doses can be lowered or omitted. A lot of men are basically unsexed by certain blood pressure medications, including the beta blockers, clonidine, methyldopa, and those containing reserpine. It is rare, but occasionally event the "water pills," ACE inhibitors, and calcium channel blockers can cause equally bad problems with ED.

Careful histories taken by a physician will often detect other drugs that can cause ED. Those include certain sedatives, tranquilizers, antidepressants, sleeping pills, certain anti-ulcer medications, and barbiturates. Elimination of the offending medication and prudent substitution of alternative medications will often help. Don't guess about your medication and stop or change the dose on your own. Let your physician know if there are prospective problems that need to be resolved.

The nutritional solution is to eat in a healthy way and avoid excess fats, salt and sodium, sweets, and alcohol. If you follow The Clinic-30 diet and get all the grains, fruits, and vegetables the program requires, your body will function more normally. That is partly because you have lost weight and feel better, but also because the antioxidants in the foods protect you from the degeneration that often speeds up in an obese person.

Alcohol is often responsible for ED, both directly and indirectly. It is recommended that alcohol consumption stop while on the active phase of The Clinic-30 Program. If you must have a drink, confine yourself to one jigger of spirits, six ounces of dry wine, or eight ounces of light beer. It may be difficult for a person to go from a lot of alcohol to a little, or none, but it's only for a relatively short time and will be worth it.

A lot of men have ED because they are drinkers. As Shakespeare wrote in Macbeth: "Drink increaseth the desire, but taketh away the performance." Some men deliberately stay up at night and drink in front of the TV, instead of going into their bedrooms. They're often afraid they won't be able to "perform" for their wives, and they drink more in frustration. I suggest a gradual cutting down of alcohol over a week's time, but not an abrupt cutoff. Some men are alcoholics and not just drinkers. Abruptly cutting off the alcohol in their case would put them in danger of D.T.'s, a potentially fatal condition. It pays to check with a physician before any radical dietary or habit changes are attempted.

Hidden diabetes is common in obese men and women and can affect sexuality in both. Diabetics often feel tired and have no energy. That is a clue for a physician that diabetes may be present. Poorly controlled diabetes is a strong risk factor for blindness, coronary artery disease, peripheral vascular disease, and cerebrovascular impairment.

I have often found that a man with ED becomes a different person once the diabetes has been identified and controlled, and some of the weight has been lost. Women whose diabetes are controlled report more energy and libido than when the diabetes was running rampant in their bodies.

Prostate problems, particularly a subclinical case of chronic inflammation of the prostate, can literally unsex a man. Prostatitis is often a disease of younger men, so any work-up should include a digital rectal exam, even for those in their early twenties. ED work-ups should always include prostate evaluations, especially in black men.

Smoking is often responsible for changes in male and female libidos. Stopping smoking for a few months can show the person just how much damage cigarettes were causing. The one drawback is that sometimes weight is gained, but even that can be stopped with exercise and careful attention to a diet.

Vitamins are not touted as treatment for ED or female sexual dysfunction (FSD), but they support the body in general and can help bring the metabolism and body function closer to normal. A good therapeutic Vitamin should help.

Caffeine is often the culprit when too much is taken in, particularly if the drink is sweetened with regular sugar. A moderate amount of caffeine is fine for most of us, but there is often a rebound exhaustion that occurs when too much sugary caffeine drinks are consumed. It is hard to enjoy sex or to function as a sexual partner if there is an overwhelming tiredness and lack of energy. Do not stop caffeine abruptly, or you could have the "mother of all headaches!" Take it slowly over a period of a week for best results.

Keep your water intake high every day. A relatively dehydrated person has little energy for lovemaking.

Women who are breast feeding often report a decreased desire for sex. One of the hormones connected with milk production interferes with testosterone production, a vital element for proper sexual desire. That's the bad news. The good news is that orgasm is more likely because another hormone present in postpartum women increases that ability.

Keep your intake of fruits and vegetables high to make sure you're getting all the antioxidants your body needs, whether you are male or female.

Level with your doctor if sexual dysfunction is present. The National Council on Aging published a survey showing that of 1300 Americans, aged 60 or older, slightly less than half of them engage in some form of sexual activity at least once a month, and about 40% of them want more sex than they are getting.

Half of the men and 12% of the women had some medical problem or problems that prevented them from having sex. Among those surveyed, 44% of the women and 13% of the men had partners with medical reasons not to engage in sexual activities. Over half of the men and women had less sexual desire, and 44% of the men and 16% of the women had been on medications that reduced their sexual drives. That is not only a shame, it's a disaster for those affected.

A PERSONAL NOTE

I feel as if we've spent a lot of time together in going over The Doctors' Clinic-30 Program, and how it can help you lose weight and keep it off.

You've discovered that your weight problem is complex, with no easy answers, but that it is not a hopeless situation.

You do need to know what to eat and how much.

You do have to follow the exchange program and watch the calorie content of certain foods and beverages.

You do have to find some reasonable way to increase your energy output, preferably through walking and other exercise.

You do need to increase your sense of self-worth and gain confidence in handling yourself in food-related situations.

You do need to change your thinking, from that of a fat person to that of a thin person.

You do need to break old habits, and form new ones.

The most important thing is not to get discouraged or overwhelmed in this process of losing fat. The multiple things you have to deal with can be handled over a period of time, one at a time.

You have to be realistic and tolerant of initial problems and mistakes as you learn these routines. Look at the entire experience of losing unwanted weight as a learning experience.

In the learning process you must take tiny bits of the overall problem and deal with each one individually. Visualize a brick wall that stands between you and your goal. You obviously can't move the entire wall out of your way at one time, but you can tear that wall down a brick at a time.

The individual "bricks" are your unique and special problems. Handle them separately. Divide and conquer! Make your experience of weight loss a pleasant one and don't take yourself so seriously if things aren't always the way they should be.

As in any learning experience, there are lessons to be studied and homework to be done. Please look upon the extra time spent as an investment in your slimmer future.

If you have to go through some discomfort in order to survive at a food-related gathering, please put up with it. A long-term goal is worth some temporary problems, and the efforts you expend today will pay off dividends in health, happiness, and the chance of a longer and more productive life.

I will be pulling for each and every one of you, along with your loved ones, and close friends who are helping you perform this vital service for yourself.

To each of you, the best of luck!

APPENDIX A

SOME RECIPES TO GET YOU STARTED

"To eat is a necessity, but to eat intelligently is an art" –
La Rochefoucauld

Here are some of my favorite recipes for slimmers. Many of these recipes were contributed by patients over the years. Others come from food companies that make sugar-free and low-calorie products. Add these to your program. I've listed how many exchanges each provides.

Once you attain your slimmer figure, experiment and read the food magazines for low-calorie food tips and recipes.

DR. COOPER'S SUPER SOUP

Take 2 green peppers, several whole tomatoes (fresh or canned), 5 large onions, 1 large head of cabbage, and 1 large celery bunch. Seasoning can be done with 8 beef or chicken bouillon cubes, or dry onion soup mix, along with other herbal seasonings as desired. Vary the seasoning for effect.

Cut and chop all vegetables into small chunks.

Boil vegetables in water with seasoning, salt and pepper to taste for at least 10 minutes. Lower heat and simmer until desired consistency of vegetables is reached. Increase or decrease water in pot while cooking to get desired thickness or thinness of soup.

The soupier it is, the better, and the more filling. This soup may be eaten in virtually unlimited amounts before, after, and between meals, plus at bedtime. You can also add certain vegetables, such as mushrooms, broccoli, asparagus, cauliflower, etc.

If there are certain vegetables you DON'T like, remove them from the soup and substitute another non-starchy vegetable.

A delicious stew can be made by putting one to two pints of the prepared mix into a crock pot with four ounces of chopped or sliced chicken, turkey, fish, shrimp, or other sea food.

The meat or meat-like food used in the preparation of the stew has to be accounted for in your daily intake figures (five or seven ounces total for the day, depending on body frame).

Let it cook all day with the appropriate spices and herbs, so that it will be ready by the evening meal.

You can also let it cook all night and have it ready to take to work in a Thermos bottle for your lunch the next day. To repeat, the meat or other protein food used in the stew is counted against the daily allotment of meat.

Those of you who must restrict your salt and sodium intake may omit the canned vegetables from the soup and use fresh or frozen only. Sodium-free bouillon cubes can also be used as seasoning when appropriate.

It's obvious that there is some caloric value in the soup, but it is relatively unimportant in the daily food intake calculations. TREAT IT AS A FREE FOOD.

POMMES FRITES A LA COOPER

Take 3 or 4 medium sized potatoes and boil them in lightly-salted water for about 9 or 10 minutes. Drain the excess water off and cut the potatoes into quarter-inch slices. Lightly dust with butter salt, garlic salt, or other seasoning to taste, and then born on a non-stick pan surface. The resulting chips, or pomme frites, are crispy and tasty, but without any added fat.

TUNA (OR SALMON) CRISPIES

Take six ounces water-packed tuna or salmon. Drain well. Mix in¼ cup finely chopped celery, 1 beaten egg, 2 teaspoons Worcestershire sauce, and salt and pepper to taste. After mixture is completely blended together, shape into two equal patties. Fry on non-stick surface without grease or oil until brown on both sides. Each crispy contains two low-fat meat portions.

PASTA SALAD

Cook three shapes of pasta until soft (not al dente). Rotini, wheels, and macaroni elbows are good in salads. Add one cup of each type of cooked pasta to a large bowl. Pasta should be cool at time of mixing. Chop three large stalks of broccoli so that no piece is larger than will fit in a teaspoon without overlapping.

Chop one large carrot into coin-shaped slices. Add two ounces of diet Italian dressing to the bowl after the chopped vegetables. Toss and mix thoroughly. Divide the mixture into three salad bowls. Sprinkle ½ teaspoon grated Parmesan cheese over the salad. Each serving is equal to two bread-pasta-cereal portions.

LOW-CAL BRAN MUFFINS

Take 3 tablespoons non-fat dry milk solids, 3 tablespoons water, 2 envelopes Sweet 'N Low, ¾ of a cored apple, ¼ teaspoon vanilla extract, 4 drops almond extract, a pinch of cinnamon, a pinch of nutmeg, and 5 to 6 tablespoons unprocessed wheat or oat bran. Put all ingredients except bran into a blender. Blend at medium speed until apple is chunky. Pour into a bowl and add bran. Whip batter with spoon and mix well. Divide batter among four cupcake holders and bake at 350 degrees for 35 minutes. Yield is four muffins. Four muffins equal a total of one low-fat milk portion and one fruit portion. Editor's Note: Although these muffins don't rise like store-bought muffins, they really taste great and are good for you.

DIET GAZPACHO

Take 1 whole onion, 1 large green pepper, 2 whole tomatoes (fresh preferred), 2 medium cucumbers (remove all seeds from cucumbers and pepper), 1 tablespoon vegetable oil, a pinch of cumin spice, 1 level teaspoon of fructose (optional), 1 tablespoon cider vinegar, 1 teaspoon lemon juice.

Chop onion, pepper, and cucumbers in food processor. Add tomatoes, one at a time, and continue processing until liquid. Add balance of ingredients and totally liquefy. Strain to remove large particles. Refrigerate and serve cold. Equal to one cooked vegetable exchange.

AU GRATIN EGGPLANT SOUP

Take a three-quart soup pot or pan. Spray PAM or other nonstick spray in pot or pan. Add one large onion and two celery stalks that have been finely chopped in a food processor, or on a cutting board. Allow the onion and celery to cook slowly until soft. Stir in two cloves of garlic, finely chopped, and cook for two more minutes. Stir in two medium-sized eggplants (aubergines), finely chopped, along with ½ teaspoon each of dried thyme and ground coriander seed.

Saute for three minutes more on low heat, then add a medium-sized red pepper that has been finely diced. Add one quart of low-sodium beef broth, chicken broth, or other low-calorie soup that has no more than 80 to 90 calories per 15-ounce can. Low-sodium stock may be used as well. Bring the mixture to a boil, cover, and let simmer for at least 30 minutes. Add two tablespoons chopped coriander leaves. Place soup in Pyrex or similar bowl; place a tomato slice on top of each soup serving. Sprinkle with liberal amounts of grated Swiss cheese, and lightly broil until cheese has melted. Serve at once. Limit this soup to one serving of six to eight ounces per day. Equivalent to about one cooked vegetable portion a day.

MOCK SPAGHETTI SAUCE

Take 1 cup vinegar, ½ cup ketchup, 1 clove garlic, 2 tablespoons Worcestershire sauce, 1 teaspoon liquid non-caloric sweetener with saccharin, 1 teaspoon dry mustard, ½ teaspoon Tabasco sauce, 1 teaspoon salt.

Mix together all ingredients and simmer 10 minutes in a saucepan. Each tablespoon contains 10 calories. You may use up to six tablespoons (three ounces) daily on pasta. Any unused portion can be stored in a closed container in your refrigerator and warmed for use as needed. Six tablespoons equals one fruit portion.

MOCK SPAGHETTI SAUCE WITH MEAT

Make mock spaghetti sauce and pour three ounces into a measuring cup. Take three ounces, raw weight, of very lean ground chuck. Brown on a non-stick surface, stirring frequently. Make sure meat is fully cooked and then drain off excess grease. Pour in three ounces of mock sauce and allow to simmer for five minutes over very low heat. Add to pasta and enjoy! Equals one fruit portion and three meat portions, plus the bread-cereal-pasta portions represented by the pasta.

OTHER PASTA SAUCES

Additional pasta sauces that are permitted on the fat-loss portion of the diet are as follows:

Newman's Own Marinara style sauce. One-half cup (4oz.) contains 60 calories, with 15 calories from fat. Consider this is a free food if you only use four ounces.

Ragu Light Pasta Sauce, Tomato and Basil Flavor. Also has 60 calories per half cup, with no fat calories from fat. This is a free food if you only use four ounces.

If you use more than a half-cup, you must count each additional four ounces as a cooked vegetable. You may use other brands if they have roughly the same caloric and fat content.

FRESH TOMATO AND BEAN SOUP

½ cup navy beans	1½ pounds tomatoes, peeled, divided, cored, and chopped
3½ cups water	¼ tsp Sweet 'N Low Liquid sugar substitute
1 tablespoon vegetable oil	½ tsp Italian seasoning
½ cup chopped celery	¼ tsp thyme, crushed
⅓ cup chopped onion	2 cloves garlic, minced, crushed
½ tsp salt	$1/_8$ tsp pepper

In saucepan, combine beans and 2 cups water; bring to a boil. Simmer about 2 minutes. Cover; set aside about 1 hour. Add additional water to saucepan to make 2 cups. Cover; simmer about 1½ hours. About 30 minutes before end of cooking time, in saucepan in hot oil, cook and stir celery, onion, and garlic about 4 minutes. Add tomatoes, Sweet 'N Low sugar substitute, Italian seasoning, salt, thyme, pepper, and remaining water. Bring to a boil. Cover; simmer about 20 minutes. Drain beans; add to tomato mixture. Cover; simmer about 5 minutes. Makes 6 1-cup servings. Exchange information: one bread-cereal-pasta; one cooked vegetable. Negligible fat.

BORSCHT

8¾-ounce cans julienne beets	10 drops Sweet 'N Low Liquid
1 tblsp vegetable	½ tsp dill
¼ cup chopped	$1/_8$ tsp pepper
1 cup shredded cabbag	¼ cup plain low-fat yogurt
1 cup beef broth	1 tblsp cider vinegar

In food processor or blender, puree 1 can beets; set aside.

In saucepan in hot oil. Cook onion about 3 minutes. Add cabbage; cook about 8-10 minutes. Add beef broth, pureed beets, julienne beets, vinegar, Sweet 'N Low liquid, dill weed and pepper; bring to a boil. Cover; simmer about 20 minutes. Serve hot or chilled, topped with yogurt. Makes four¾-cup servings. Exchange information: two cooked vegetables.

OAT BRAN MUFFINS

1½ cups low-sugar bran cereal crumbs

5 packets Equal

½ cup raisins

1 tablespoon baking powder

1 cup skim milk

2 eggs, beaten

1 tablespoon oil

2 tablespoons Mott's unsweetened apple sauce

Use half low-sugar bran cereal with NutraSweet and half oat bran cereal.
Line microwave muffin pan with paper baking cups. Crush cereal and combine dry ingredients. In a separate bowl, combine moist ingredients. Mix dry and moist ingredients, let stand for about 5 minutes. Stir. Fill muffin cups¾ full. Microwave on medium (50 percent) for 6 minutes. Exchange information: one bread-cereal-pasta group;½ fat portion.

MOLDED PERFECTION SALAD

1 envelope unflavored gelatin	½ cup minced celery
¼ cup cold water	½ cup shredded red cabbage
1½ cups unsweetened orange juice	½ cup shredded green cabbage
1¼ cups shredded carrot	1 tblsp minced chives

In small saucepan, sprinkle gelatin over cold water. Let stand 1 minute. Heat, stirring constantly until gelatin dissolves. Remove from heat, stir in orange juice and Equal. Chill about 25 minutes or until slightly thickened. Stir in vegetables and chives. Pour into 1-quart mold, sprayed with nonstick coating; chill about 4 hours, or until set. Unmold to serve. Makes 8½-cup servings. Exchange information:½ fruit portion.

YOGURT CUCUMBER SALAD

1 medium cucumber, thinly sliced	4 packets Equal
½ cup thinly sliced red onions	½ tsp salt

157

½ cup plain low-fat yogurt   1/8 tsp pepper

Combine cucumber and onion slices in a bowl. Combine remaining ingredients and pour over slices. Toss. Serve immediately.

Each of the 4½ cup servings has 36 calories and may be considered as a free food if only one is eaten. If two servings, count as one vegetable.

CRISP SWEET SLAW

Slaw:	Dressing:
4 cups shredded cabbage	¼ cup cider vinegar
½ cup chopped onion	½ cup apple juice or cider
1 cup chopped green pepper	3 tblsp vegetable oil
	8 packets Equal
	1 tsp celery seed
	1 tsp dry mustard
	1 tsp salt
	$\frac{1}{8}$ tsp pepper

Combine slaw ingredients. Whisk together dressing ingredients. Pour over slaw, toss to blend. Refrigerate until served. Exchange information: one fat exchange and one free vegetable per serving. One serving is equal to one cup.

PEACH GINGER FROTH

Serve in cold, frosted glass. Dip glass in water and chill in freezer 15 minutes, or until frosty.

Ingredients	One Serving
Skim milk	½ cup
Peeled, pitted and sliced fresh peaches	¼ cup
Almond extract	$\frac{1}{8}$ teaspoon (tsp)
Ginger powder	$\frac{1}{8}$ tsp
Equal	1-2 packets

Ingredients	One Serving
Ice	2-3 cubes

Combine all ingredients in blender. Blend on high for 30 seconds, or until light and frothy. Pour into tall, thin glass and serve. Makes an 8-ounce serving. Exchange information:½ nonfat milk and½ fruit.

GRAPEFRUIT APPLE ZINGER

Freeze grapefruit or apple juice in an ice cube tray and serve with this drink.

Ingredients	One Serving
Unsweetened grapefruit juice	¼ cup
Unsweetened apple juice	¼ cup
Bitters	1-2 dashes
Equal	1-2 packets
Club Soda	¼ cup

Stir together grapefruit and apple juice, bitters, and Equal in a tall glass. Add club soda and enough ice to fill glass. Stir and serve. One fruit exchange.

STRAWBERRY CHOCOLATE SHAKE

Ingredients	One Serving
Fresh or Unsweetened frozen strawberries	½ cup
Skim Milk	½ cup
Unsweetened cocoa powder	2 tsp
Equal	2-3 packets

Combine all ingredients in blender. (Add 3-4 ice cubes if using fresh strawberries.) Blend on high for 30 seconds or until smooth and creamy. Pour into tall glass and serve with straw, Exchange information:½ nonfat milk and one fruit, per serving.

THE BASIC SHASTA OR DIETRITE SHAKE

1 (12-oz) can Diet Shasta or DietRite fruit drink (any flavor)

⅓ cup instant nonfat drymilk 1 portion fresh fruit

1/8 tsp vanilla extract

Salt to taste

1 cup coarsely crushed ice (about 12 cubes)

Combine all ingredients in top of blender. Blend on high until frothy. Makes 1 quart. Exchange information: one fruit and one nonfat milk. Choose fruit to complement soda flavor used, such as berries, orange, pineapple, or cantaloupe. If you want more fruit in each quart of mixture, account for it in your daily diet calculations.

APPENDIX B

RESOURCES FOR SLIMMERS

Here are some sources of information, equipment, and other items you might find helpful during your weight-loss program.

The addresses and phone numbers were accurate as this book went to press, but please understand that addresses and phone numbers do change from time to time. I have used many of these products and sources of information, and so have many of my patients.

VITAMIN SUPPLEMENTS

The vitamin formula I wrote is now available to the public. Order through our office and we will ship the vitamins directly to your home. For more information on prices and ordering, contact:

Marietta Office
1234 Powers Ferry Road
Suite 104, Marietta GA 30067
Office: (770) 952-7681
Fax: (770) 952-8688
www.dietdrtom.com
www.drfatakhov.com

FOOD SCALES

Try your local office supply and use a postal scale, or check with your nearest department store and see if they have food scales. You want the type that will let you weigh even semi-solid foods.

WALDEN FARMS SALAD DRESSINGS

These salad dressings are tasty and convenient to use, with both bottles and individual packets available in several flavors. Call or write the company for more information. You can order directly through the company, or get the name of a store near you that carries these products.

Walden Farms
P.O. Box 352
Linden, NJ 07036
Phone: (908) 925-9494

MORE LOW-CAL RECIPES

Some of the recipes in this book were courtesy of the following companies. For more great recipes, contact them directly.

Equal Consumer Relations (makers of NutraSweet and Equal)
P.O. Box 2986
Chicago, IL 60654
Phone: 1(800) 323-5316

Shasta Beverages
Customer Relations
26901 Industrial Blvd.
Hayward, CA 94545
Phone: (510) 783-3200

Cumberland Packing Corp. (makers of Sweet 'N Low)
Dept. HHR
60 Flushing Ave.
Brooklyn, NY 11205
Phone: (718) 858-4200

You can also get more information on low-calorie foods from:
The Calorie Control Council
www.caloriecontrol.org

Weight-Control Information Network. (WIN)
WIN is a service of the National Institute of Diabetes and Digestive and Kidney Diseases of the National Institutes of Health
www.niddk.nih.gov/health/nutrit/nutrit.htm

Food and Nutrition Information Center, U.S. Dept. of Agriculture
www.nal.usda.gov/fnic

BARIATRIC PHYSICIANS

I have been a proud member and former president of the American Society of Bariatric Physicians (ASBP) for over 45 years. We have members in every state in the U.S., Canada, and parts of Mexico. If you feel like after you're done with this program that you need professional help and want caring, knowledgeable medical professionals then consider going to the ASBP website, www.asbp.org

You may ask for the doctors in your area and get their addresses and phone numbers. The A.S.B.P. neither endorses, nor do they oppose, the diet and the diet book you are reading.

BIBLIOGRAPHY

Hertog, M. G., Bueno-de-Mesquita, H. B., Fehily, A. M., Sweetnam, P. M., Elwood, P. C., & kromhout, D. Fruit and Vegetable Consumption and Cancer Mortality in the Caerphilly Study. Cancer Epidemiology, Biomarkers & Prevention, 5, 673-677.

Key, T. J., Thorogood, M., Appleby, P. N., & Burr, M. L. Dietary habits and mortality in 1000 vegetarians and healthy conscious people: results of a 17 year follow up. British Medical Journal, 313, 775-9.

Kendall, A., Olson, C. M., & Frongillo, E. A. Relationship of hunger and food insecurity to food availability and consumption. Journal of the American Dietetic Association, 96, 1019-1024.

Larsen, T. M., Dalskov, S., Baak, M. V., Jebb, S. A., Papadaki, A., Pfeiffer, A. F., et al. Diets with High or Low Protein Content and Glycemic Index for Weight-Loss Maintenance . The New England Journal of Medicine , 363, 2102-2113.

Appel, L. J., Moore, T. J., Obarzanek, E., Vollmer, W. M., Svetkey, L. P., Sacks, F. M., et al. A Clinical Trial Of The Effects Of Dietary Patterns On Blood Pressure. The New England Journal of Medicine , 336, 1117-1124.

Heidelbaugh, J. J. Management of Erectile Dysfunction . American Family Physician, 81, 305-312.

Shamloul, R., & Ghanem, H. Erectile dysfunction. The Lancet, 381, 153-165.

About Us. (2013, January 1). Retrieved, from http://www.asbp.org/about.html

Seger JC, Horn DB, Westman EC, Lindquist R, ScintaW, Richardson LA, Primack C, Bryman DA, McCarthy W, Hendricks., et al.Obesity Algorithm. American Society of Bariatric Physicians. Retrieved, from www.obesityalgorithm.org

www.ingramcontent.com/pod-product-compliance
Lightning Source LLC
Chambersburg PA
CBHW050221270326
41914CB00003BA/522